Psychiatric Interviewing and Assessment

Second Edition

D1235885

Psychiatric Interviewing and Assessment

Second Edition

Rob Poole

Professor of Social Psychiatry, Centre for Mental Health and Society, School of Social Sciences, Bangor University, Bangor, United Kingdom

Robert Higgo

Senior Lecturer in Social Psychiatry, Bangor University, Bangor, United Kingdom; Honorary Consultant Psychiatrist, Mental Health Liaison Team, Wrexham Maelor Hospital, Wrexham, United Kingdom

CAMBRIDGE
UNIVERSITY PRESS

CAMBRIDGE
UNIVERSITY PRESS

University Printing House, Cambridge CB2 8BS, United Kingdom

One Liberty Plaza, 20th Floor, New York, NY 10006, USA

477 Williamstown Road, Port Melbourne, VIC 3207, Australia

4843/24, 2nd Floor, Ansari Road, Daryaganj, Delhi – 110002, India

79 Anson Road, #06–04/06, Singapore 079906

Cambridge University Press is part of the University of Cambridge.

It furthers the University's mission by disseminating knowledge in the pursuit of education, learning and research at the highest international levels of excellence.

www.cambridge.org
Information on this title: www.cambridge.org/9781316614037
DOI: 10.1017/9781316676554

First published 2006
Second edition 2017

Printed in the United States of America by Sheridan Books, Inc.

A catalogue record for this publication is available from the British Library

Library of Congress Cataloging-in-Publication data
Names: Poole, Rob, 1956–, author. | Higgo, Robert, 1952–, author.
Title: Psychiatric interviewing and assessment / Rob Poole, Robert Higgo.
Description: Second edition. | Cambridge, United Kingdom ; New York, NY : Cambridge University Press, [2017] | Includes bibliographical references and index.
Identifiers: LCCN 2017023048 | ISBN 9781316614037 (alk. paper)
Subjects: | MESH: Interview, Psychological – methods | Personality Assessment | Mental Disorders – diagnosis | Physician-Patient Relations
Classification: LCC RC480.7 | NLM WM 143 | DDC 616.89/075–dc23
LC record available at https://lccn.loc.gov/2017023048

ISBN 978-1-316-61403-7 Paperback

....

This second edition is dedicated to the memory of Dr Kevin White and Richard Marley, who provided us with the inspiration and support we needed to write about psychiatric skills.

Contents

Preface

We are living through difficult times, and psychiatric practice is changing rapidly. During the preparation of this book, two ageing psychiatrists sat at a kitchen table, drinking coffee, and discussing the state of their profession, their country and the world. One said to the other:

'You know, for millennia, men of our age have sat around tables like this, complaining that since they were young, everything has gone to the dogs. It's just our luck that this time it really has.'

Despite continued declarations of the imminent demise of our profession, we believe that psychiatry has a strong intellectual and clinical tradition that has a great deal to offer people with mental illness, and that it will continue to flourish in a recognisable form long after the current turmoil in the world and in the health professions has passed.

This book aims to help mental health professionals to develop core clinical skills in psychiatric interviewing and assessment. We have tried to produce a book that we would have found helpful at the beginning of our careers. The content is relevant to a range of mental health disciplines, including nursing and social work, despite a strong focus on psychiatric practice. We have aimed to write in a readable and authentic style, and working as psychiatrists is what we know best. We have not attempted to write from the viewpoint of other disciplines. Responses to the first edition suggested that this decision was correct, and we hope that this second edition will be helpful to practitioners of other professions.

This book is not about treatment, pharmacological or psychological. It is not about highly specialised assessments. It is about broad-based generic skills, which form the foundation of all other clinical interventions.

The book assumes the level of knowledge of psychiatry necessary to qualify as a medical practitioner or as a mental health nurse in the UK. The book has a general orientation towards community psychiatric practice. British psychiatry has a strong tradition of pragmatism and theoretical eclecticism whilst aspiring to follow the evidence base. This book follows that tradition. Where we have expressed opinions, or have taken a controversial point of view, we have tried to clearly indicate this. We have kept referencing to a minimum, as we believe it undermines readability.

The book is intended to be a guide to clinical practice. It is built around situations that are recognisable from clinical experience. We have used clinical vignettes to illustrate principles throughout the book. We have taken great care to make these realistic. We have not used true stories. Our patients and colleagues may feel that they recognise themselves in the vignettes. If so, they are mistaken. If some stories seem familiar, it is because there are recurrent themes in clinical practice.

We have 65 years of clinical experience between us: in deprived inner city areas; in rural Wales; in assertive outreach; amongst the homeless; in acute inpatient care; and in general hospital liaison psychiatry. We have learned that the most important objective in psychiatry is to get alongside patients. This does not mean doing whatever patients want. It means working in an alliance whereby the patient is supported by the clinician to find a route to recovery. The task is relational, embedded in everything that goes on between the professional and the patient. It cannot be neglected while some technical task is completed.

Furthermore, it can only be achieved if the clinician has an awareness of the importance of context and is able to understand the patient's point of view. It is true that this perspective demands some effort from the clinician early in the relationship. However, we have found that, overall, it takes less effort to do psychiatry well than to do it badly.

In writing the two editions of this book, we reflected long and hard on our own clinical practice. We hope that this has not resulted in a text that is idiosyncratic and anecdotal, but that other experienced clinicians will recognise the processes and dilemmas that we have identified. The book has five overarching and interrelated themes, which are important in clinical practice. These are:

- Process: assessment is not a battery of questions to be asked, but a process between two people. Attention to process optimises assessment and creates the foundations for a therapeutic alliance.

- Patient-centredness: understanding the patient as a person and understanding their subjective experience of their illness is an essential perspective in evaluating psychopathology, risk and other issues. We explore the patient's experience of the interview through examination of the separate agendas of the professional and the patient. Resolving the tensions and conflicts between these agendas is a key task for the clinician.

- Context: we explore the impact of the patient's psychological and social context, the context of the interview and the professional's psychological and social background as important factors that can assist or interfere with assessment.

- Hypothesising: it is often suggested that assessment consists of information gathering and mental state examination followed by diagnosis or formulation. In fact, experienced clinicians operate by forming hypotheses and testing them throughout an assessment. This is an efficient, flexible and critical process. There are significant pitfalls. If you fail to recognise that you are likely to form impressions very early in interviews, then those impressions are not easily challenged. A conscious awareness of the hypothesising process makes for better assessments.

- Clinical scepticism: this is that essential critical and independent-minded quality that is shared by all good doctors. It leads to a questioning of psychiatric orthodoxy and to an awareness that patients, their families and their friends all provide information that is affected by their subjective standpoint.

The most useful psychiatric books are read as much for pleasure as for self-improvement. This book is intended to be a light read, but its objective is serious. We felt that the process of writing the first edition made us more reflective, self-aware clinicians. We hope that this second edition proves relevant and helps other clinicians to avoid the mistakes we made along the way.

Acknowledgements

We were delighted and surprised that the first edition of this book was well received in the UK, the USA and beyond. We had a great deal of help from friends and colleagues in preparing that original text, including Dr Sue Ruben, Gordon Kennedy, Dr Theresa McArdle, Dr Richard Barnes, Gill Strong, Richard Marley, Dr Kevin White and Dr Michael Göpfert.

In preparing a second edition, we have expanded the scope of the book to accommodate some changes in the way that psychiatrists work. There is new material on neurodevelopmental assessments, on assessing adolescents and on rhetorical interviews, amongst other topics. We have adapted the text to the arrival of DSM-5, and we have tackled issues over the use of psychometric instruments in clinical practice. Ignoring wise counsel, we have rewritten most of the old material.

The task was daunting for a number of reasons. Firstly, there is the risk of following success with failure. Secondly, clinical practice has changed dramatically in the years since the first edition was published. Capturing current practice without being overly negative was quite a challenge. Finally, we have, through an unusual set of circumstances, both become clinical academics. In our earlier existence as inner city community psychiatrists, we were often dismissive of our academic colleagues. As we have written, we have internally heard the mocking voices of our younger selves, amused that two academics would presume to write a book about clinical skills. We have been fortunate to have significant assistance in the task, especially from Professor Catherine Robinson, Dr Sue Ruben, Dr Theresa McArdle, Dr Daniel Poole and Professor Peter Lepping. We have particularly valued their assistance in preparing the substantial amount of completely new material. We have retained the striking cover image from the first edition, painted by Sue Ruben.

What Am I Trying To Find Out Here?

There is an unavoidable problem at the heart of the work of all health professionals. The practice of medicine and allied professions is increasingly based on empirical science, generating interventions that are essentially technological and standardised. These technologies may be psychological, social or biological (or involve a combination of these modalities). The scientific-technological has to be applied in the context of patients' lives, which are rich in complexity and ambiguity. At its simplest, no matter how efficacious a drug may be, it cannot work if the patient does not take it. The factors that make patients reluctant to accept advice may appear irrational to clinicians, but they are highly relevant to patients. No one can be expected to accept an intervention unless they are reasonably certain that the balance of the cost–benefit equation will lead to a positive change that is relevant to the quality of their life.

Much of this book is concerned with the development of the fundamental skills of forming and maintaining relationships with patients in order to deploy technologies without causing harm. This first section, however, is about a simultaneous, more technical task: developing a formulation, including a diagnostic understanding of the patient's problem. This is based on history taking and mental state examination.

The objective of this section is to understand what you are looking for during assessment, and to explore some of the problems associated with this technical task.

Diagnosis

The Medical Model

'The medical model' is a puzzling concept. For many years, there appeared to be a consensus that the medical model as applied to mental disorder was a bad thing, and for the most part only the most convinced biological psychiatrists were prepared to defend it. However, it is far from clear what the term actually means. Sometimes it is used to mean the dominance of doctors amongst the mental health care professions. On other occasions, it refers to institutional models of care. Most frequently, it is used to characterise a sterile, de-humanised, genetic-pharmacological stance that does exist, but which cannot be reasonably described as the mainstream of psychiatry. A telling definition of 'the medical model' was given to us by a clinical psychologist many years ago, which is that it is anything that doctors do. This definition has the virtue of being logical.

In recent years there have been efforts to reassert the importance of medical skills and perspectives in mental health care (e.g. Craddock et al. 2008; Burns 2013). We are happy to defend one type of medical model, which remains in robust good health, despite decades of sustained criticism and attack from a wide variety of sources. We recognise that it has limitations and contradictions, but it is the de facto model of mental health care across the world, and it is not going to go away. Furthermore, it has some strengths. So far, no one has come up with a better alternative that could plausibly be expected to improve our ability to help people with mental disorder.

Few people could work in health care without being embarrassed or angered by the actions of doctors from time to time, either because of individual shortcomings or because of institutional self-interest. No profession could defend itself on the basis of the activities of its worst practitioners. The underlying model of medicine is the application of empirical science to help people in the context of their lives and environments. The scientific and human tasks are of equal importance. When medicine runs into trouble, it is usually because the scientific and the human tasks have become disconnected.

Out of this medical model have sprung pharmacological and surgical treatments, and also the whole of public health, including understanding of the role of hygiene, sanitation, nutrition, housing and inequality. The origins of psychotherapy and of social intervention to improve the health of the population lie within medicine and have a basis in this paradigm.

Where medicine has tried to impose crude technologies on patients, it has usually been based on poor or even pseudo-science, which is a betrayal of the fundamental task of the profession. The strength of medicine, and therefore the medical model, is its ability to understand problems at multiple levels simultaneously and to intervene in helpful ways that are informed, but not dominated, by scientific empiricism.

Diagnosis is a component of the medical model. It is a concept that unequivocally belongs to medicine and to the general medical approach to the understanding of human suffering. Embedded within the idea of diagnosis is an implicit assumption that symptoms, signs and natural history group together to form syndromes; that such syndromes can be understood at a physiological level; and that this can lead to the discovery of pathological processes and underlying causations.

The movement of diagnosis from syndrome, to physiology, to pathology, to causation, has underpinned a substantial proportion of all progress in medicine. It has been particularly effective in understanding infectious diseases and finding treatments and preventive measures for them. It has underpinned the substantial progress that has been made in responding to the global AIDS pandemic and the Ebola epidemic in West Africa.

The same process has sometimes been effective in understanding mental disorders. In the nineteenth century, 'general paralysis of the insane' (a type of neuro-syphilis) and some forms of complex partial epileptic seizure were regarded as part of an undifferentiated syndrome of 'insanity'. Now they are well understood and can be treated with reference to underlying organic pathologies and physiological processes. In modern times, this process led to the identification and better understanding of Lewy body disease from amongst the dementias of old age.

Categorical Diagnosis in Psychiatry

Notwithstanding these examples, and despite recurrent claims that psychiatric diagnosis in general is about to move on from the level of syndrome to neurophysiology, it must be acknowledged that there is little evidence that we are anywhere close to this. Despite extensive research effort into the major syndromes (such as schizophrenia, bipolar affective disorder and depression), consistent and coherent underlying physiologies, pathologies and causations remain elusive. The lack of clear biological causations is probably not just the consequence of inadequate scientific knowledge. No matter how far we progress scientifically, some psychiatric problems are unlikely to prove to have a primarily biological basis (although as scientific materialists we assume that all psychological activity must have associated brain activity).

When considered overall, psychiatric diagnosis is heterogeneous, embracing a wide diversity of disorders. This includes dementias (which definitely have a basis in coarse brain disease), psychoses (some of which probably have a basis in either brain dysfunction or subtle structural abnormalities), personality disorders (which are probably in large part developmental problems as a consequence of childhood adversity) and psychological reactions (which arguably lie within the range of normal human experience). The biological reductionist approach on its own is unlikely to be useful in understanding or managing many of these problems, no matter what scientific advances occur.

A primary concern of patients is the development of effective, safe, tolerable and user-friendly treatments, and here progress has been relatively good. However, few treatments in psychiatry are specific to diagnosis. In the main, our treatments are effective for particular symptoms. Antipsychotic drugs are useful in treating delusions and hallucinations, irrespective of diagnosis, and cognitive–behavioural therapy (CBT) has been shown to be useful in treating virtually every major mental disorder, provided the symptoms make the person either anxious or depressed. Some modern critics of psychiatric diagnosis (e.g. Bentall 1992; British Psychological Society 2013) have argued that the whole nosology is illogical and unscientific, and should be abandoned. It is argued that we should focus on specific psychological problems rather than on diagnoses. Whilst this stance has utility, it ignores the secure knowledge that we do possess, which has important practical and scientific implications. We do have an excellent understanding of the ways in which symptoms group together, the course that such syndromes generally follow, some of the ways in which these disorders develop and the factors that tend to relieve or exacerbate them.

Until the 1970s it was difficult to defend psychiatric diagnosis, as, frankly, the nosology was a total mess. A series of well-known international studies (e.g. Cooper et al. 1972) used operational definitions to show that the prevalence of the major psychoses was remarkably similar in different countries. Nonetheless, national statistics showed wide variation, as psychiatrists of different nationalities had entirely incompatible definitions for the same disorders. Consequently there was no common international psychiatric language. At that time, psychiatric diagnosis could be criticised for lacking basic semantic validity. As a consequence, idiosyncratic diagnostic systems and diagnostic concepts in various countries came under critical scrutiny.

One of the repetitive errors of psychiatry has been to base diagnosis on supposed, but unproven, causations. A key example was the distinction in the UK between 'endogenous' and 'reactive' depression. Endogenous depression was said to arise from within the person without psychological or social antecedents (probably owing to a hereditary factor). It was said to be severe and characterised by biological symptoms. Reactive depression was less severe and closely related to the person's circumstances. Vulnerability to reactive depression was believed to be related to social stress and personality. Unfortunately, the neat distinction fell apart when studied closely (e.g. Kendell 1976). The presence of biological symptoms turned out to be a reflection of the severity of depression, and stressors were shown to be equally important at either end of the severity spectrum. Not only did symptoms fail to cluster into two groups, it was also more difficult than expected to demonstrate that anxiety and depression were separate syndromes.

The development of the International Classification of Diseases, Tenth Edition (World Health Organization, 1992) (itself influenced by the development of successive Diagnostic and Statistical Manuals in the USA) elevated psychiatric diagnosis to the level where categories had some basis in demonstrable syndromes. This classification (universally known as ICD-10) is a multi-axial diagnostic system with operational criteria for various diagnostic categories. It has been shown to have face validity and clinical utility. It allows psychiatrists to share an international scientific language that can be readily understood by reference to an accessible and understandable glossary. Indeed, the ICD-10 glossary is essential reading for psychiatrists in training. It is well written, clear and includes explanations of the nature of the categories. However, there are new controversies over psychiatric nosology.

ICD-10 is almost 25 years old, and ICD-11 has been under preparation for some time. In 2013, the American Psychiatric Association published the fifth edition of DSM, DSM-5 (APA 2013). Amongst many other changes, this version of DSM is not a multi-axial classification but a dimensional one. This document is intended for use in the USA, where it is ubiquitous. One important use is by health care insurers to determine remuneration for psychiatric treatment.

NHS England has devised a system of 'diagnostic clusters' for a similar purpose, in order to introduce 'payment-by-results' into mental health care. Although there is widespread support for incentivising better outcomes for patients, the mental health diagnostic cluster system is deeply flawed. Psychiatrists working in England are unlikely to be able to ignore the Mental Health Care Clustering Tools associated with this system, as they determine the amount of cash that returns to the organisation for treating each patient. Tools to determine tariff payments should not be mistaken for diagnostic instruments. They are actuarial tools for estimating appropriate cost of treatment. They have to be endured rather than reified.

In the media, DSM-5 is frequently described as 'the psychiatrist's Bible'. This is wildly inaccurate. It has nothing in common with a sacred text. Far from being unassailable to criticism, controversy has raged about DSM-5. There are allegations that it has proliferated the number and range of psychiatric diagnoses, pathologising normal psychological processes; that it lacks proper scientific validity; that the committees that developed it were overly influenced by the pharmaceutical industry; and that there is excessive secrecy over how decisions were made. At first, the American Psychiatric Association and the US National Institute of Mental Health appeared to disagree over the value of DSM-5, although they have said subsequently that this was based upon a misunderstanding of the two organisations' positions.

Everyone appears to agree that there are significant problems with current diagnostic systems. Despite an aspiration to an evidence-based nosology, we retain diagnoses that take putative causation, rather than symptom clusters, as their starting point (e.g. post-traumatic stress disorder). Given the state of development of psychiatry as a science, our diagnostic schedules are provisional, and they will be revised and replaced in due course. They are useful as long as you recognise the limitations to their application.

A diagnostic manual is like a cross between a dictionary and a map. Diagnosis provides a model for understanding the relationship between different disorders. It tells patients and clinicians where an individual's mental health problem lies within the whole psychiatric terrain. It tells you little or nothing about the person and their life. Like a dictionary or a map, diagnosis does not necessarily tell you very much beyond generalities.

Beyond Diagnosis: Formulation

Psychiatry has recognised the inadequacies of using categorical diagnosis in isolation for a very long time. After the Second World War, British psychiatry emphasised the need to develop a 'formulation' of each case, largely under the influence of Sir Aubrey Lewis (the first Professor of Psychiatry at the Institute of Psychiatry in London). A formulation was a detailed understanding of the contextual factors, biological, psychological and social, which had predisposed, precipitated and perpetuated a patient's disorder. The concept of formulation implicitly acknowledged that diagnosis on its own was of limited usefulness in helping people. The importance of the formulation was that it gave a far more detailed understanding, and could guide treatment. The term fell from use in the UK quite suddenly when two psychiatrists conducted research on the concept (Hollyman and Hemsi 1983). They asked British psychiatrists (and psychiatric postgraduate examiners) what should be included in a formulation. There was no general agreement. As a consequence, the term was dropped from British postgraduate examinations, and was replaced by the term 'assessment'. This had an identical function to formulation. No doubt if a further study had been conducted, there would still have been no general agreement. Box 1.1 sets out some key elements of formulation.

BOX 1.1 Some Components of Formulation

Wherever it is possible, formulation should be a collaborative process with the patient, which should include:

- A summary of the patient's core problems
- An indication of how those problems relate to one another
- An indication as to why the patient presents now, with these problems, in this form
- A plan for treatment/intervention

Formulation has made something of a comeback in the past decade. It is mentioned in the curriculum for Membership of the Royal College of Psychiatrists, as a skill in the Health and Care Professions Council regulations for psychologists, and it is used in cognitive–behavioural, systemic, psychodynamic, personal construct and narrative therapies. The British Psychological Society has claimed that the ability to formulate a case is unique to clinical psychologists (Division of Clinical Psychology 2010), but we have to disagree. It is a skill common to all professions that attempt to help people with mental disorders on the basis of scientific knowledge.

In our opinion, the difficulty in pinning down exactly what should be included in a formulation reflects the futility of operationalising the obvious. The diversity of factors that may be important is such that it is impossible to make a single statement as to what should be included and, more importantly, what should be left out. Assessment has to include the patient's concerns and those pressures, weaknesses and strengths operating in their lives, because these are the factors that are most important in finding a path to recovery. Ways of understanding mental disorder that avoid meaning at a human level are essentially sterile and are of very limited helpfulness. It is self-evident that disorders that affect feelings, thinking and behaviour have an important dimension of meaningfulness: not obscure or unconscious meaning, but a more accessible emotional and practical meaning. Whilst it may be useful at times to think of mental disorders as arising within the brain or the mind, the true location of these problems is in people's lives.

Alternatives to Formulation

ICD-10 attempts to deal with complexity by having five axes (see Box 1.2). This does allow a more comprehensive, operationally defined description of a problem, and does clearly allow for the fact that personality disorder is a risk factor for mental illness, not a mutually exclusive diagnosis. However, the system is only useful administratively. In the clinical situation, a list of categorically arranged problems, stripped of all context and meaning, is of little help.

An alternative approach to both formulation and multi-axial classification is the use of the problem list. This was developed, for the most part, by clinicians with an interest in CBT, and it closely follows the intellectual traditions of that approach. The model is widely used in the clinical assessment schedules that have become prevalent since professions other than psychiatry have taken on the task of initial assessment.

It is not suggested that problem lists replace diagnosis. The problem list is a tool, sitting alongside diagnosis and providing a way of breaking complex difficulties down into a series

---

BOX 1.2 ICD-10 Axes

Axis I: Mental disorder (e.g. syndromic mental illness)
Axis II: Developmental disorder (e.g. personality disorder)
Axis III: Intellectual impairment (e.g. learning disability)
Axis IV: Physical disorder
Axis V: Psychosocial problems

BOX 1.3 A Problem List

Mrs A, a 53-year-old woman with late-onset paranoid schizophrenia
   Problem 1 Auditory, tactile and olfactory hallucinations and paranoid delusions regarding neighbours
   Action 1 Consultant psychiatrist to arrange treatment with antipsychotic medication
   Problem 2 Reluctant to take medication owing to limited insight into the nature of the problem
   Action 2 Community mental health nurse to carry out insight directed or concordance therapy
   Problem 3 Conflict with neighbours owing to arguments based on paranoid delusions
   Action 3 Social worker to organise rehousing for patient and her husband
   Problem 4 Psychosis worsened by worries over debts
   Action 4 Social worker to organise referral to welfare rights worker to maximise state benefits and to assist with debt management
   Problem 5 Conflict with daughters, who have been unable to comprehend their mother's behaviour
   Action 5 Community mental health nurse to conduct sessions with the family

---

of discrete identifiable problems, each of which can be tackled with reference to an action plan. A problem list might look something like Box 1.3.

Problem lists have an attractive commonsense quality, and lend themselves to clear monitoring of progress. Most clinicians use some form of problem list to organise interventions, even if the list is not formalised in this way. There are potential pitfalls to the approach. Breaking problems down can lead to a loss of long-term and thematic perspectives, in other words breaking things down too much can drain the meaningful connections between individual problems. As far as possible, problem lists need to be developed with the patient, not imposed on them, as they can turn into a paternalistic and disempowering programme. Some clinicians feel that they overlook the importance of more subtle, but important, factors arising out of relationships with individual clinicians that can contribute to (or impede) recovery.

There are many other approaches to the task of producing a concise, coherent account of the important features of a patient's disorder in the context of their life. Like many experienced clinicians our preference is for a narrative, a story that draws all the threads together so that we, and the patient, can understand what has happened to them, set in a chronological framework. This preference may simply reflect our personalities, but we believe that it has real advantages. We find that a narrative is easier to remember, and is easier to convey verbally to other professionals. Even in an age of assessment proformas it is important to find an approach to formulation that works for oneself and one's patients.

> **BOX 1.4** The Diagnostic Hierarchy in Psychiatry
>
> 1. Coarse physical brain disorder
> 2. Psychotic disorder (schizophrenia, bipolar affective disorder, persistent delusional disorder, depression with delusions)
> 3. Personality disorder
> 4. Depression without delusions
> 5. Anxiety states

Diagnostic Uncertainty

At the end of an assessment interview, it is conventional for the psychiatrist to write out a differential diagnosis. This is a list of the main diagnostic possibilities, ranked in order of decreasing likelihood. It may include both diagnostic alternatives and additional diagnoses. In the UK, differential diagnosis is pragmatic. It should include only what is plausible, not every conceivable possibility, no matter how unlikely. In some countries, exhaustive thoroughness is highly valued, but the whole British medical tradition rejects this as unfocused and unhelpful.

The differential diagnostic process reflects the fact that even the most thorough assessment is unlikely to generate diagnostic certainty. Diagnostic uncertainty can persist for years, though usually it can be resolved reasonably promptly. An excessive impatience to make a firm diagnosis leads, over time, to patients accumulating multiple diagnostic labels, which is confusing for everyone. Diagnostic uncertainty has to be managed, as it cannot be eliminated.

The commonest cause of uncertainty is lack of information, which itself plays against the backdrop of the diagnostic hierarchy in psychiatry (see Box 1.4). The diagnostic hierarchy has to be considered, no matter what system of diagnosis and formulation is used. The principle is that conditions higher up the hierarchy can cause symptoms of conditions lower down the hierarchy. The most important point is that all psychiatric disorders, no matter how typically they may present, can be caused by underlying physical disease. This means that there is *always* a degree of uncertainty, as physical disease is not always detectable, even with the use of the full range of physical investigations.

A weakness of multi-axial approaches is that they cannot properly accommodate the diagnostic hierarchy, which leads to multiple diagnoses where there is, in fact, one problem with multiple consequences.

In some respects, the hierarchy is not 100 per cent reliable. One could argue at length as to whether personality disorder should appear in the hierarchy at all. It is included mainly because quite convincing presentations of personality disorder can turn out to be due to other disorders. For example, apparent anti-social personality can arise in the context of chronic low-grade hypomania. This diagnostic error would be likely to occur in the absence of comprehensive information, but we all work in an imperfect world, where significant decisions must sometimes be made without as much information as you would like.

Hypotheses and Cumulative Certainty

A theme of this book is hypothesising. We believe that it is a process that underpins all good mental health practice, though it is rarely articulated. Diagnoses, and much else, exist as

> **BOX 1.5** Schneider's First Rank Symptoms of Schizophrenia
>
> - Delusional perception
> - Third person auditory hallucinations, including running commentary
> - Somatic hallucinations
> - Disorders of the possession of thought (hearing one's thoughts spoken out loud, thought insertion, thought withdrawal, thought broadcasting)
> - Passivity experiences (thoughts, actions and emotions experienced as literally under the control of an external agency)

> **BOX 1.6** Alcohol Dependency Syndrome
>
> - Salience/primacy of alcohol consumption
> - Craving/compulsion to take alcohol
> - Tolerance of the effects of intoxication (or loss of tolerance at a late stage)
> - Repeated episodes of withdrawal symptoms
> - Relief drinking to control withdrawal symptoms ('eye-openers')
> - Narrowing of drinking repertoire
> - Repeated reinstatement of drinking after abstinence

clinical hypotheses that must be continuously tested. When something happens, or when information comes to light, which does not fit with usual patterns, clinical hypotheses have to be reconsidered.

Related to this is the concept of cumulative certainty, the process by which a particular diagnosis or formulation becomes increasingly (but not necessarily absolutely) certain. This is codified in some particularly tricky diagnostic areas. Long before operationalised diagnostic criteria emerged, psychiatrists had difficulty in clearly distinguishing first-episode schizophrenia from other psychoses and severe affective disorders, creating uncertainty over prognosis. Kurt Schneider developed the concept of 'first rank symptoms' (Schneider 1959), which is to say a group of symptoms that are particularly characteristic of schizophrenia (see Box 1.5). Whilst all of them can arise in other disorders, the more that are present, the more likely it is that the patient is suffering from schizophrenia. Contemporary research criteria are more reliable, and modern nosological systems do not rely upon them, but first rank symptoms continue to have a clinical usefulness.

Similarly, there was long-standing controversy as to where the boundary between normal drinking and alcoholism lay, together with difficulties in defining severity of alcohol dependency problems (see Box 1.6). Edwards and Gross devised 'the alcohol dependency syndrome' (Edwards and Gross 1976) with explicit reference to Schneider's first rank symptoms. Rejecting a clear boundary between normal and problem drinking, they identified seven key features. The more the patient displays, the more severe the problem. After 40 years, this remains a helpful clinical tool.

The emergence of Early Intervention Services for psychosis has reinforced the importance of hypothesising and cumulative certainty. There is a body of evidence that shows that the longer the gap between the onset of psychotic symptoms and the commencement of treatment, the worse the outcome for the patient. It is impossible to be certain about causality; people with more insidious onset of psychosis and with more 'negative' symptoms are known to have worse outcomes, and these factors may also delay presentation for treatment. Nonetheless, it would be hard to dispute that early intervention in psychosis seems like a good idea, especially as psychotic illness tends to commence in the late teens and early twenties, which is an important and formative period in everyone's life. It is possible that long durations of untreated psychosis are intrinsically damaging.

In order to intervene early, people must be treated when they have prodromal symptoms of psychosis rather than the full syndrome. To wait for people to get ill enough to meet diagnostic criteria would be counterproductive. However, not everyone who has psychotic symptoms will go on to develop psychosis. Some isolated symptoms are common in the general population. A quarter of everyone experiences auditory hallucinations (or possibly an even higher proportion of the population). This means that judgements about whether an Early Intervention Service should treat a particular individual, and when to discontinue treatment, have to be made on the basis of uncertainty. Working hypotheses have to be reviewed and tested regularly. It is much easier to know what to do once a diagnosis has emerged, but the purpose of Early Intervention Services is to prevent people from developing full-blown psychosis. This is a clinical challenge, but it is also a challenge to the way in which psychiatrists conceptualise mental illness.

Stigma

In psychiatry, diagnosis has a profound effect upon the patient. Many patients feel that the social stigma attached to their diagnosis is more problematic than the symptoms of the illness itself. 'I have diabetes' or 'I have asthma' are statements that have implications for an individual's lifestyle and even their life expectancy. Such diagnoses can cause significant problems, for example, in obtaining life insurance at a reasonable premium. However, these statements, when made in a social setting, have only a limited impact on the sufferer's relationship with the rest of the world. The disclosure 'I have bipolar affective disorder', on the other hand, is likely to cause an irrevocable and unwelcome shift in a social relationship. Even if the diagnosis is later withdrawn because it has turned out to be wrong, the patient's previous relationship with the rest of the world is not restored. 'At first they said I had thyrotoxicosis, but apparently I haven't after all' has an entirely different impact to 'At first they said I had schizophrenia, but apparently I haven't after all'. These problems of social stigma cannot be dismissed or ignored. Patients justifiably complain that a psychiatric diagnosis is a burdensome label, which leads to loss of autonomy and to social marginalisation.

As a consequence of this, some clinicians are reluctant to make the most socially stigmatising diagnoses at all. Many are reluctant to share such diagnoses with their patients and their families. This solves no problems, and can amount to a betrayal of the fundamental duty of truthfulness. Patients and families frequently complain of a lack of diagnosis. Once reasonable care has been taken to make a full assessment (which can take some time), a clearly explained diagnostic formulation, including an explanation of such ambiguities and uncertainties as exist, is essential. It allows people to understand what has happened to them, to access as much information as they need and to secure assistance from non-health care agencies such as the voluntary sector and self-help groups. All of these can be crucial in helping people to regain control of their lives.

Over many decades euphemisms have been introduced to try to reduce stigma. Attempts to replace 'mental handicap' with 'intellectual disability' and 'mental illness' with 'mental distress' are just two recent examples. If patients prefer these terms, we should respect their choice, but objectively speaking, there is little evidence that they have achieved much in reducing stigma. Stigma rests not in words, but in social attitudes, themselves based on ignorance and fear. In the UK, politicians and the media have tended to exacerbate stigma with regard to serious mental disorders by an expedient recourse to crude and inappropriate stereotypes. As clinicians we have three duties with respect to the stigma attached to the diagnoses we make: to recognise that diagnosis tangibly affects patients' lives; to eliminate stigmatising attitudes from our own practice; and to be part of a wide alliance to combat stigma in the general public. At the most basic level we should recognise that patients are not, for example, schizophrenics, but people with schizophrenia.

Main Points in This Chapter

1. Diagnosis has a role in understanding mental disorder, but it has problems and limitations.
2. Diagnosis is insufficient on its own to allow us to understand patients' problems.
3. No person can be defined or fully described by a diagnosis.
4. The problems with psychiatric diagnosis are also evident in other areas of medicine, though they may be less immediately obvious.

Chapter 2

History

What is the Point of History Taking?

The whole of the practice of psychiatry rests upon access to a reliable and comprehensive history. No one can expect to treat any patient safely without a good understanding of how they have come to develop this problem at this time. Without knowledge of their lifestyle, concerns, strengths and weaknesses, attempts at intervention are likely to be clumsy and inappropriate. Obtaining a full history is by far and away the most important task in psychiatric assessment. It is of considerably greater value than technically more complex tasks such as mental state examination, cognitive assessment or physical investigations, though each of these is important in its own right. Mental state examination, for example, is essentially a snapshot located in a moment in time. Consequently, if too much reliance is placed upon it in making a diagnosis, it can be misleading. Mental state examination needs the context provided by history in order to be meaningful.

All mental health professionals make assessment errors from time to time. In our experience, errors most often occur because the history is inadequate. You might suppose that this usually happens when patients first come into contact with mental health services, as decisions often have to be made before comprehensive information is available. In fact, at this stage, professionals are usually aware of the ambiguities caused by lack of information, and tend to be appropriately cautious as a consequence. Problems more frequently arise when patients have been in contact with services for a while. Continuing history taking is sometimes neglected because the person is 'well known to the service'. Sometimes, parts of the patient's history have not been properly understood or have been forgotten; and sometimes, something new and important has happened, but the professionals miss it because no one thinks it necessary to ask. It is self-evident that no one can ever know everything about another person. The objective, therefore, is to collate an adequate history, but to bear in mind that the task is never really complete.

History taking is not a passive process of information collection. It is an active and continuing process, which involves understanding and organising information. This chapter is not about the process of obtaining a history, which is dealt with elsewhere in this book. Here, we are concerned with the information that needs to be collected and how it should be organised. The emphasis and detail needed varies in different situations, but the main components of an adequate history are, for the most part, invariable.

Proformas have proliferated in clinical practice, mostly embedded in myriad computerised record systems. Forms can provide an *aide-mémoire* for history taking, but they are a very awkward method of keeping records. There is a perverse incentive to cover parts of history with a generalisation, rather than detail. It can be very difficult to retrieve information from proformas, whether paper or digital.

Proformas can dictate the way that an interview is conducted, leading the interviewer to interrogate the patient and impose excessive control over the direction of the discussion. Needless to say, we do not like assessment proformas much, as we feel that they cause more problems than they solve. Leaving aside practical considerations, they remind us of the pre-Second World War admission sheets which could be found in the case notes of long-stay patients in old-fashioned mental hospitals when we started our careers. These were elderly people who lived barren, institutional lives for decades, having been first admitted as young people. The admission sheets, on heavy foolscap paper with copperplate handwriting and a faded photograph, seemed to signify the reduction of the patient's life to an administrative procedure.

Despite these unpleasant resonances and limitations in practice, assessment proformas are part of modern health care culture. Proformas must be completed properly. In our opinion, it is best to interview in the traditional patient-focused way, and to fill in the forms afterwards. This is time consuming, but no one can conduct an effective psychiatric interview whilst staring at a computer screen.

General Considerations

Box 2.1 sets out the underlying structure of a psychiatric history. A straightforward initial assessment might generate a history following this general pattern, with information under each of the headings. Various authorities have suggested that histories should be set out in different orders, but the headings rarely differ. This is the structure that we have found most useful in general adult psychiatric practice. It lends itself to later amendment and expansion. We rarely sequence interviews in exactly this way. As we discuss later, this is a structure for organising histories, not for sequencing interviews. In particular, history taking and mental state examination are not, in the real world, fully separate tasks, though they are recorded separately.

The structure covers all aspects of the patient's life, and forms a kind of abbreviated biography. Very few people think about themselves and their lives in this structured

---

BOX 2.1 The Basic Structure of a Psychiatric History

- Reason for referral
- History of presenting problem
- Psychiatric history
- Family history
- Childhood history
- Educational history
- Occupational history
- Sexual and reproductive history
- Medical history
- Social history and daily routines
- Substance misuse history
- Forensic history
- Pre-morbid personality

biographical way. Consequently, constructing a chronology is an essential task when organising the information that you are given. Gaps in chronology, in other words, periods when it is not clear what was happening in the person's life, are important. They demand further enquiry. Histories should either be organised around the patient's age at the time, or the date, whichever the patient finds easier. Without this, gaps will go unnoticed. Combinations of date and age are confusing, and are to be avoided if at all possible.

There is a general principle that it is far more illuminating to ask people about the tangible than about the abstract. For example, asking a patient why their marriage broke up invites a general, and uninformative answer, such as 'I wasn't very happy in the marriage and we drifted apart', whereas asking what happened, about the events that provoked the split, focuses on the particular, and is more likely to reveal reasons. Although you are concerned with the patient's feelings, what actually has happened in their life is the basis of a good history.

Reason for Referral

In psychiatry, very few things happen suddenly. Most people have been struggling with their problem for months, or even years, before they finally come for help. How they came to be sitting in front of you is relevant both to the here and now of the interview, and in understanding the overall situation. Did they come of their own volition, or did they come under duress? Why have they come now, rather than last week or a month ago? Why did the referrer think the patient needed assessment? What events provoked the request for assessment? The answers to these questions reveal the concerns of the patient and the concerns of those around them. It is especially important to elicit and record this information when people are assessed out of hours or in emergency situations, not least because it can be impossible retrospectively to find out what has gone on.

History of the Presenting Problem

The point here is to understand what is worrying the patient, and to understand how the problem has developed. What symptoms and behaviours are most concerning the patient and those around them? When did they start? Did any events or stresses seem to provoke or exacerbate the problem? What effect is the problem having on the patient's daily functioning? Can they cope with their job? Are they looking after their children properly? Are there changes in their motivation to do things that they usually enjoy or feel to be important? What have their family and friends done in response to the problem?

Are they sleeping well? If not, they may be unable to drop off to sleep, or they may wake early. Sleep may be light with recurrent waking. Their sleep pattern may have reversed, with napping by day and wakefulness at night. Sleep is hard to assess, as broken sleep is often experienced as continuous wakefulness, which can lead people to believe that they are not sleeping at all. It is important to find out when they go to bed and when they rise. What do they do when they cannot sleep? On the one hand, getting up for a cup of tea or coffee, or a cigarette, worsens sleeplessness; on the other hand, people who lie awake all night in darkness and silence are probably sleeping more than they realise.

Has their eating pattern changed? Are there corresponding changes in their weight? A lot of people do not weigh themselves regularly, but nearly everyone notices when clothes become tighter or looser.

Is their concentration affected? The question is not always meaningful to people who do not have to attend to complex tasks or absorb a lot of information as part of their occupation. For many people, poor concentration is experienced as forgetfulness. Some relatively banal activities demand a fair degree of concentration, including video games and following the plots of soap operas or police procedurals. Questions about changes in concentration should not be an abstract enquiry, but need to relate to those tasks that arise regularly in people's lives.

Some would include a general question regarding mood and suicidal thoughts here, if they have not arisen as part of the description of the main problem. In the sequence of the interview they are often dealt with next. We discuss them under mental state examination, as that is where they belong structurally. However, what does belong here is any history of self-harming behaviour, the circumstances in which it occurred, what the patient had expected to occur as a consequence and what did actually occur as a consequence. Assessment of suicidality is dealt with in Chapter 19.

Is there anything that the patient has found that helps how they feel? Has their family doctor (GP), or anyone else, tried to treat them? Did it make any difference? If medication was prescribed, did they take it? Did they experience side effects?

Psychiatric History

This includes both whether the patient has ever seen a mental health professional before, and whether they have experienced symptoms (whether similar to the current symptoms or not) prior to the current episode. Previous treatments and their outcome (including whether the patient experienced them as helpful) are obviously relevant. It is especially important to ask about previous psychiatric admissions, the length of the stay and whether the patient was subject to legal compulsion. Dates, locations and names of professionals are important in obtaining old records, which normally requires the patient's explicit and written consent.

Family History

Though it is relevant to ask if other family members have suffered from mental health problems, family history is much more than this. It is important to ascertain the structure of the patient's family of origin. This includes parents' current ages, occupation and the quality of the patient's relationship with each of them. Where parents have separated or one or both parents have died, the parent's and the patient's ages at the time are important reference points for the rest of the history. Ages of siblings, current relationship and a brief outline of their circumstances are also important. Where family structures are complex, it can be helpful to draw a schematic family tree (see Box 2.2).

We have found that many people confuse step-siblings (i.e. non-biological relationships with the offspring of step-parents) with half-siblings (i.e. those who share one parent). Equally, there is confusion between step-parent (the partner of a biological parent) with foster parents (adults who care for children on a temporary basis, often, but not always, as a job). Both of these are confused with adoptive parents (adults who take on full legal responsibility for children but are not biologically related to them). Each of these relationships has different implications, and drawing a clear distinction between them can be important.

BOX 2.2 Example of a Family Diagram

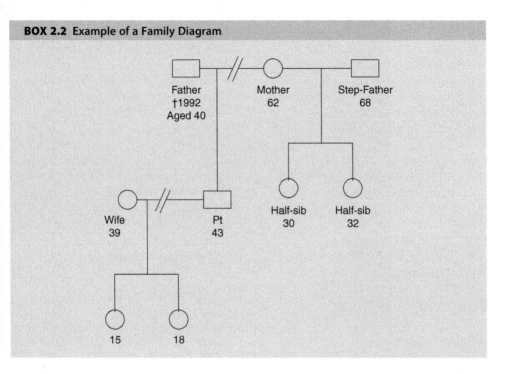

Childhood History

Whilst some people can spontaneously give a detailed account of their childhood, this is rarely possible for people who have experienced a disrupted and disturbing childhood. Whilst this is not surprising, given that it is difficult to make sense of an unhappy childhood as you live through it, these are actually the childhood histories that are most important to understand. It is conventional to ask about developmental milestones (ages of first walking, talking, reading, etc.), but in our experience, hardly anyone knows the answer unless there has been marked delay. Similarly, we were taught to ask about 'childhood neurotic traits', such as thumb-sucking and nail-biting, but no one has ever explained to us why they are important. These behaviours are widespread in the population and they are of little significance. It is, however, worth asking about bed-wetting, as this can persist to adulthood, with a major impact on self-esteem.

What are more important are early losses and separations, any history of violence in the home and the patient's recollection of periods of persistent childhood unhappiness. The general rule about concentrating on the specific is particularly true here. Statements that a childhood has been unhappy tend to mean that the patient felt different to other children. They reflect a comparison. You need to know about events and family behaviours. This may involve direct questions about specific types of difficulties. Questions around these issues will frequently uncover histories of emotional or physical abuse. Direct questions about childhood sexual abuse are usually best dealt with as part of sexual history, though people increasingly make spontaneous disclosures in psychiatric interviews, often as a consequence of being distressed by coverage of the issue in the media.

Educational History

Educational histories are best divided into the main educational phases, which in the UK are primary school, secondary school and higher education. The types of school attended are relevant, together with changes of school and reasons for them. Peer relationships at school, especially any history of bullying or being bullied, disciplinary problems, truancy (absence without parental/carer knowledge) and school refusal (absence with knowledge/complicity of parent/carer) should all be subject to enquiry if they are not volunteered. Academic attainment, including grades of any qualifications, should be ascertained. Where there is evidence of educational problems, it is worth directly asking about special schooling and referrals to child and adolescent mental health services or educational psychologists. Under these circumstances, it is important to ask about literacy. Problems with reading and writing are far more widespread than is generally acknowledged, and can occur in otherwise intelligent people. Illiteracy tends to be accompanied by shame. 'Have you ever had problems with reading and writing?' captures the full range of difficulties, past and present. 'Can you read and write?' has an entirely different connotation and invites a misleading and defensive reaction, as illiteracy is rarely absolute.

Occupational History

For most people, occupation (like relationships and reproduction) is one of the main reference points by which they structure their understanding of their life. A significant proportion of people with severe mental disorders have little or no experience of work, which is a major contributing factor in their social marginalisation. Where patients have an occupational history, the detail needed depends on how frequently job changes have occurred. If a middle-aged man has worked in the building industry, then the nature of the work is often casual and temporary, and he is unlikely to remember details of each job. Asking whether he has ever been sacked, or has lost jobs due to ill health, is more relevant. Less frequent changes, including promotions and redundancies, can be important in more settled employment histories. Recurrent disputes with employers or workmates, or episodes of being bullied, are important. They may not be volunteered unless you ask whether the patient enjoyed the job, and if not, why not.

Sexual and Reproductive History

The first issue in any sexual history is sexual orientation. This may be volunteered or become obvious early in interviews, but not always. A significant proportion of insecure heterosexual men become surprisingly upset if you ask them if they are gay. They take the question as an affront to their masculinity, as they hope that their heterosexuality is some-how self-evident. Consequently, the question is best put by asking the patient whether they are heterosexual, rather than asking them to deny homosexuality. Few gay people are offended by the question put this way round. The question cannot be avoided and it becomes more difficult to ask later on. Asking the question becomes more offensive to the homophobe after you've had a chance to get to know them, as it becomes a deeper assault on their sexual identity (which for most homophobes is conflicted or ambivalent).

Apart from this, you are trying to understand the person's history of serious (and therefore usually sexual) relationships; the quality of their current relationship, and what has gone wrong in past relationships. This may or may not lead to exploration of actual sexual problems. Age of puberty and of first sexual contact is generally relevant. Age of menopause and whether relationships are still sexually active is relevant in older people.

It is normally appropriate to ask a general question as to whether the person has had unwanted sexual experiences as a child or as an adult. Asked in this way, histories of childhood sexual abuse and rape may be volunteered. It is important not to press people into early disclosure of bad sexual experiences, as making such a forced disclosure to a stranger can be traumatising and unhelpful. The point is to indicate that the issue is available for discussion. Many people make disclosures in later interviews after initial denials, having had a chance to think about it.

The modern concern with sexual abuse has tended to reduce focus on the importance of reproductive histories. In all cases, you want to know about patients' children, their current circumstances and so on. Occasionally, this can be important in identifying child protection concerns. However, lost pregnancies, whether through miscarriage or medical termination, are important events. They are often overlooked unless you ask women how many times they have been pregnant before asking how many children they have. Similarly, single men can lose contact with their children by alienated partners, which is often a source of major distress.

Medical History

Current physical health problems and past illness, including hospital admissions and operations, should be recorded in detail. Patients should be asked what medication they are taking; drug names and dosages should be recorded, if possible. This is different from asking what they are being prescribed. Lists of medication in referral letters only tell you what the referrer thinks the patient is taking. The entire general population is not very compliant with intended drug regimes, and any doctor who thinks that their patients usually follow their instructions with regard to drug treatments is not asking patients about their use of medication in the right way. People should be asked about allergies; although this will elicit information about a host of non-allergic adverse responses to all kinds of agents, it is the only way to ensure that one knows about potentially life-threatening reactions.

Social History and Daily Routines

Social history is about the person's daily life at present. What type of housing do they have? Who owns the accommodation? Who is in the household? This may not be immediately obvious. Do they have friends and a social life? Have they given up social activities or contact with friends lately? Are there financial problems? If so, how did debts arise, how much do they owe (i.e. hundreds or thousands of pounds) and are they getting any help with this? What are their interests or hobbies? Some people deny having any hobbies or interests, in which case it can be illuminating to ask what newspaper they read (if any), what television programmes they like and their taste in books, films or music.

Daily routines reveal a lot about a person's functioning. Simple questions, such as 'How do you spend your time each day?' and 'How did you spend your time before you became ill?' will usually elicit the information. Where a patient cannot, for whatever reason, answer these questions, it can be helpful to get them to describe a 24-hour period hour-by-hour, usually through describing the previous day.

Substance Misuse History

Substance misuse is extremely common amongst people with mental health problems. Whilst some types of substance misuse can be the primary cause of mental ill health, more commonly it is a dysfunctional strategy to deal with feeling bad, which unfortunately tends to exacerbate the problem. The media, policy-makers and providers of mental health services have been preoccupied with the problem of drug misuse for years. Whilst the problems caused by recreational drugs are serious, this preoccupation has tended to obscure the dangers associated with alcohol use, which is far more widespread. Heavy alcohol use can have considerably worse effects on a person's mental health than occasional use of drugs.

A key challenge in taking a substance misuse history, and in understanding it, is that patterns of substance misuse are constantly changing. There is a wide range of psychoactive substances available. The traditional categorisation of psychoactive substances into opiates, hallucinogens, CNS stimulants and CNS depressants has utility, but it is too crude to fully understand the effects of all of the substances that are commonly misused. Cannabis, for example, has effects that fall into three of these four categories. Young adults commonly use 'legal highs'. These are more accurately known as 'new psychoactive substances' (NPS), as they are not necessarily legal, and 'high' may not accurately describe their effects. A huge international trade in NPS has developed over the Internet, and the main consequence is that people often do not know what it is that they have taken, which may include older drugs rebranded, drugs with extensive and unusual effects that are hard to categorise (such as ketamine) and substances with toxic effects on humans that are only vaguely understood.

Tobacco, alcohol and recreational drugs are not the only substances that are widely available. Other substances are misused, often by people who do not conform to drug or alcohol misuse stereotypes. The misuse of prescription drugs (especially benzodiazepines) is common. Over-the-counter medicines are also misused, especially those containing codeine. Caffeine tablets are remarkably potent, as are proprietary cough medicines. Solvent misuse still occurs, primarily, but not exclusively, in young teenagers. The cult of female thinness is matched by a corresponding male preoccupation with muscle bulk. The use of anabolic steroids and other less reliable anabolic agents is commonplace in gym culture. Herbal remedies are generally perceived as 'natural' and therefore safe, but they can be potent, and toxic in large doses.

Specific communities use substances that are unfamiliar to the rest of the population. For example, ghat (or khat) is a shrub that grows in East Africa. The leaves are chewed by men in the Somali and Yemeni communities. It has much the same effect as amphetamine, and causes similar problems with heavy use. It is illegal throughout North America and Europe, including the UK (from 2014). There are other examples of less well-known abusable substances.

It is neither practical nor desirable to ask every patient about every potentially abusable substance. Questions about less common types of substance misuse are triggered by clues, and largely rest upon the professional's knowledge of the patterns of substance misuse. A young man who reports going to the gym regularly should be asked about steroids, but there is little point in posing the same question to a frail older person. This is not the same as allowing your assumptions to replace appropriate questions. Not all heavy drinkers look like 'alcoholics', and there are people with alcohol problems even amongst devout religious communities that prohibit alcohol use completely.

Practically speaking, obtaining a substance misuse history rests on a combination of routine questions and pursuing clues from history and mental state examination. For example, it is quite difficult to accidentally burn the end of your nose, unless you use crack cocaine (commonly turned to vapour using a flame; the crack and the flame are held in the direct vicinity of the nose). A burn to the tip of the nose invites a direct question. Similarly, it is reasonable to assume that anyone who attends an appointment smelling of alcohol has a drink problem, no matter how vehemently this is denied. Drinking before a serious meeting breaks a social taboo, and reflects the salience of drinking. The fact that this may be an attempt to control the anxiety generated by the meeting does not alter the fact that it is problem drinking. A smell of alcohol, lingering from the night before, reflects very heavy consumption, and one can safely assume that someone who claims they had 'a couple of glasses of wine' is either fooling themselves or has a very loose definition of 'a couple'. If someone close to you has suggested that you drink too much, you almost certainly have a problem. A conviction for drink-driving invariably indicates an alcohol problem.

In routine histories, you should ask how much tobacco the patient uses, and this is, of course, straightforward. Alcohol is more difficult. The probe 'Do you drink alcohol?' is less useful than 'How much do you drink?' or 'How much alcohol do you take?' This follows the general principle that, when asking about common behaviours which are socially embarrassing or seen as shameful, it is usually best to avoid structuring questions in such a way that there is an element of confession in the answer. Framing the question around the assumption that the person does drink is unlikely to offend the non-drinker and makes it easier for the drinker to open up. Similarly, the probe 'How much cannabis do you use?' is useful with people under 60. Cannabis use is common and attracts relatively little social opprobrium, notwithstanding widespread publicity about an association with schizophrenia. Cannabis can cause quite severe problems in its own right, but it is likely to be perceived as innocuous.

Whilst the majority of people who use cannabis do not use other drugs, nearly all serious drug users use cannabis. People who have never used cannabis are highly unlikely to regularly use other illegal drugs. Confirmation of cannabis use therefore opens up more detailed questioning about other drugs. However, in the case of drug use, the more direct approach can be effective. The question 'Have you ever used drugs?' does usually seem to generate a truthful answer, though it can shock people who are socially conservative. Contrary to their reputation, the vast majority of drug users are disarmingly frank about their habits. It is, nonetheless, important to ask 'anything else?' as they describe their substance misuse, as the substance of most concern to the user may not be the only substance relevant to their mental well-being.

People who drink too much, on the other hand, have a strong tendency to minimise their consumption. This is related to a key feature of alcohol misuse, denial. Drinkers tend to mislead themselves. It is necessary to pin people down, including quantities and which branded drinks they prefer. It is easy to ascertain the strength of these on the Internet. Falls and symptoms of withdrawal are significant where alcohol consumption is heavy.

We have dwelt on substance misuse histories at some length, both because they are important and also because they present real difficulties. Box 2.3 sets out a menu of questions, not to be used as a rigid schema but to illustrate some useful lines of enquiry. No history taking technique is completely reliable and you have to maintain a relatively high level of suspicion that there may be an undisclosed substance misuse problem, no matter how well you know the patient. It is worth pointing out that older people can develop

BOX 2.3 A Menu of Specific Questions in Drug and Alcohol Histories

Alcohol

- At what age did you start drinking?
- Exactly how much did you drink yesterday, and at what times?
- Which brand, and what strength, of beer/cider do you drink?
- Do you drink wine as well? Do you ever drink spirits?
- Exactly what did you drink on your worst day this month?
- How much do you spend on alcohol? Where does the money come from?
- Have you ever been convicted of drink-driving?
- Do other people think your drinking is a problem? Do you agree?
- Has your tolerance increased? Do you shake or retch in the mornings?
- Have you ever tried to give up drinking? What made you try?
- Have you had falls or accidents when drunk or suffered from memory blackouts?
- Have you ever had a fit or hallucinations when you stopped drinking?
- What about drugs?

Drugs

- At what age did you start using drugs?
- What drugs have you ever used, and what do you use now?
- How do you pay for it? Do you owe money to a drug supplier?
- Have you ever injected drugs?
- Have you ever had a bad drug experience? Or had withdrawal symptoms?
- Do you think drugs cause you any problems?
- Which of the following do you use? Heroin, methadone, pharmaceutical opiates, benzodiazepines, cocaine, crack-cocaine, amphetamine, ketamine, LSD, magic mushrooms, ecstasy (and its analogues), cannabis, exotic drugs (e.g. khat).
- What about alcohol?

alcohol problems for the first time in their lives, and that this may not be evident to those around them. You have to ask.

Forensic History

This refers to the patient's history of criminality. Overall, people with mental health problems are no more likely to offend than the general public, though career criminals who become mentally ill often become less adept at their art and are caught more frequently as a consequence. Set against this, a substantial proportion of the population has at least one conviction. Men are more frequently convicted than women, and much more frequently imprisoned.

The probe 'Have you ever been in trouble with the law?' is fairly neutral, and seems not to offend the law-abiding. Not all prosecutions result in a conviction, and asking only about the patient's criminal record may miss important patterns of offending. Ideally, one should record the date of each prosecution, the exact offence (if the patient can remember), the circumstances leading to the prosecution and any penalty imposed. Some people have enormous criminal records for petty offending, in which case it may be more relevant to ask about convictions outside of their usual pattern, for example whether a habitual shoplifter has any convictions for aggression. People who have convictions should be asked about similar behaviour that has not come to the attention of the criminal justice system, in other words, how often they have got away with it.

Pre-Morbid Personality

Medical students are taught to ask patients what kind of person they are, or were before they became ill. This is worth asking, as it tells you how the patient sees themselves at present and the effect of their problem upon them. In the assessment of personality, however, it can be seriously misleading.

Personality development is important in psychiatry. It is the psychological substrate within which everything else occurs. In every case, the psychiatrist has to make an assessment of the patient's personality, and of the extent to which behaviours that are presently evident are due to illness, as opposed to personality factors. The assessment of personality is difficult and requires some skill. For example, you need to be able to infer personality characteristics from history. 'Pre-morbid' personality is a misnomer, suggesting that personality is submerged or destroyed once mental illness takes hold. This is far from the truth. Personality remains an active shaper of behaviour even in the most severe and continuous mental illnesses, though the expression of underlying personality can be changed considerably by illness.

The main objection to calling this part of the history taking schema 'pre-morbid personality' is not semantic, but practical. Hardly anyone can give an accurate account of their own personality. A remarkable proportion of anxious and troubled people will report their normal personality as 'happy-go-lucky' or even 'bubbly' in the face of evidence of chronic unhappiness. Few people understand how others experience them. No one ever describes oneself as 'insufferably pedantic' or 'touchy to the point of being paranoid', though such personalities are common enough. Full assessment of personality is dealt with in Chapter 18.

The only real point in asking patients what they are like is that their answer reflects their self-esteem and their concerns about themselves. However, this is usually evident from other parts of the interview. We feel that this section should be retitled 'Usual self' and alongside it, in every case, an assessment of personality should stand alongside diagnosis, demanding just as much care and attention in arriving at conclusions. To leave personality assessment as a postscript to history taking seems to us to be entirely misconceived.

Main Points in This Chapter

1. An adequate history is the most important part of psychiatric assessment.
2. Taking a structured psychiatric history requires the interpretation and organisation of information.
3. The standard schema of psychiatric history taking is not a guide to the structure of the interview itself.
4. History taking is never a completed task, no matter how long you have known the patient. No one can ever know everything about another human being.
5. We do not like assessment proformas or the concept of 'pre-morbid' personality, but we strongly suspect that both of them will outlive both of us.

Chapter 3

Mental State Examination and Psychopathology

The ability to observe and empathically understand other people is the key attribute of a good psychiatrist. It is always important to understand a patient's preoccupations, concerns and experiences. Mental state examination is a specific task, a formal and structured exploration of the features that are evident as the patient sits before you. The idea of mental state examination is derived from the distinction in medicine between history (the account that the patient gives of *symptoms*) and examination (looking for *signs* that can be demonstrated at the bedside). The parallel is not an exact one, as mental state examination includes exploration of experiences that are intrinsically subjective, and which may not be occurring in the here and now.

Mental state examination requires an understanding of descriptive psychopathology. This is a huge subject, and an exhaustive account of it is beyond the scope of this book. Here we explore the general principles of mental state examination. We will attempt to clarify those psychopathological issues that most commonly cause confusion.

The Limitations of Traditional Descriptive Psychopathology

Generations of British psychiatrists were trained to follow an approach to descriptive psychopathology that is most clearly set out in the first two editions of Frank Fish's seminal book *Clinical Psychopathology* (Fish and Hamilton 1985) (the 2007 third edition (Casey and Kelly 2007) is, in effect, a completely different book, but there is a modern standard textbook that continues in this tradition: Oyebode 2015). It is an approach that has been criticised on a number of different grounds (e.g. Bentall 2003), including that it is overly influenced by the clinician's values. Most clinicians recognise that it has limitations and that it is in need of revision. Unfortunately, there is no generally accepted new approach that could replace it, despite extravagant claims by some that they have devised alternatives (e.g. Kinderman 2014).

As a consequence of functionalisation of care and the spread of assessment by proforma, there has been a tendency to replace the traditional model of trying to understand what the patient has experienced with simply recording what the patient has said. This is unequivocally a step backwards. It is important that clinicians master the traditional model, even if it is then rejected for a newer approach to subjective experience. Descriptive psychopathology is an important clinical tool and its strengths and limitations must be understood.

We have significant doubts about some elements of traditional teaching on psychopathology. Here we must issue a warning. A good knowledge of conventional psychopathology is an absolute necessity if you want to pass postgraduate psychiatric examinations.

We would not want our scepticism to lead others into failure in exams that we safely passed long ago.

It is generally accepted that Karl Jaspers was the father of psychopathology. In a brief career as a psychiatrist, he wrote 'General Psychopathology' (Jaspers 1913) before going on to a career as an existentialist philosopher (an occupational route that few career advisers recommend these days). His influence is still felt through his use of phenomenology as a method of understanding the experience of mental illness, and in the emphasis on form rather than content of psychopathology.

Phenomenology is a philosophical tool for exploring subjective experience. The idea is that it is insufficient to simply note that the patient has said something that sounds like an abnormal experience. Quite apart from anything else, variations in the ability to express oneself mean that you have to be quite sure that patients are describing psychopathology rather than simply using an unusual form of words. The presence of psychiatric jargon in the vocabulary of the population at large (for example, 'I'm feeling paranoid', meaning 'I'm feeling self-conscious') makes this all the more important.

In practical terms, the phenomenological approach attempts, so to speak, to get inside the other person's head and examine the emotions and thoughts that form a mental context for each individual item of psychopathology. Having imagined yourself into the patient's frame of mind, you can then start to explore the form and content of each idea or experience. For example, is an idea primary (arising *de novo*) or secondary to an emotion or another idea? Is a belief not only false, but also held with an abnormal resistance to reason, in which case it may have a delusional level of fixity (bearing in mind that we all believe some things which are palpably not true)? Is an experience or idea understandable if you take into account the context or is it non-understandable and bizarre (in which case it may have a schizophreniform quality)? The patient's subjective experiences are compared against a set of psychopathological definitions and criteria, and then categorised accordingly.

Clearly, this approach rests on the clinician's ability to empathise and imagine. The extent of this ability varies between clinicians. Whilst it improves with time, experience also teaches that mental phenomena often do not fall into discrete typologies. For example, the definitions of delusions and obsessional thoughts are quite different, but they can mutate into each other. Some people seem to experience intermediate or mixed phenomena. Some describe experiences that seem to lie entirely outside of the standard psychopathological categories.

In recent decades, cognitive–behaviour concepts have been applied to a wide variety of mental disorders, including schizophrenia, and there is significant research interest amongst clinical psychologists in psychopathology. As a consequence, a range of fundamental psychopathological concepts, such as the fixity of delusions and the non-understandability of schizophreniform symptoms, has been challenged. The service user movement, under the banner of Recovery, has forced us to critically re-evaluate many aspects of psychiatric practice, including our understanding of psychopathology. For example, 'hearing voices' embraces a far wider range of human experience than previously realised (e.g. Romme and Escher 1993), though there is sharp disagreement as to whether 'voices' experienced by people who are not psychotic represent *forme fruste* psychosis or whether these are distinct experiences of an entirely different nature. For both scientific and clinical purposes, the presence of psychopathology does not necessarily imply the presence of a mental illness, though mental illness does, by definition, always involve experiencing psychopathology.

In daily clinical practice, the identification of psychopathology can be highly dependent upon the clinician's expectations, and upon their initial assumptions about the nature of the patient's problem. For example, when uncooperative and difficult people are admitted to hospital, it is tempting to decide hastily that they have a personality disorder. Psychopathology is then interpreted through the filter of this assumption. However, a range of presentations of psychosis, from low-grade hypomania to awkward and fatuous presentations of hebephrenic schizophrenia, can look very similar to personality disorder. The psychopathology can only be recognised if you can distance yourself from the personality disorder assumption.

Expectations always exist. No clinician can go into a clinical assessment free from any idea about what is likely to be the problem. One of the reasons that we emphasise hypothesising throughout this book is that it provides a way to avoid being misled by assumptions. You can achieve this by making your assumptions explicit as hypotheses and testing them.

The problem of prior assumption is equally true with regard to the recognition of phenomena that do not fit into a well-defined psychopathological type. When confronted with a conflict between what the patient says and what the textbooks say, doctors the world over have a disheartening tendency to place an unquestioning faith in textbooks. As a consequence, there is a reluctance to identify ambiguous phenomena as such, and a tendency firmly to classify them into an inappropriate category.

In the history of psychiatry, there are a number of examples of whole types of psychopathology emerging or disappearing. Whilst this may sometimes reflect real changes in the incidence of certain types of problems, it is sometimes an artefact of changing clinical fashions and expectations. For example, catatonic states were once amongst the commonest of psychotic presentations. For many years it was generally believed that such symptoms were no longer seen in the Western world, except amongst people of Asian and African origin. Fink and Taylor have strongly argued that this is not true (Fink and Taylor 2003), but that as diagnostic fashions changed, the characteristic features of inaccessibility, mutism, posturing, over-arousal and undirected excitement came to be interpreted differently. The distinction does matter, because the usual treatments for psychotic symptoms do not work well for catatonic symptoms, and there are other treatments which are much more effective.

In the light of all this, the use of psychopathology has to be seen as being similar to the use of diagnosis. They are tools that should not be reified. We need descriptive psychopathology as a way of organising what we observe, but if we put faith in it as an adequate way of wholly describing our patients, it will let us down badly.

Doing Mental State Examination

There is more than one way of doing mental state examination. Finding a personal style and a range of probe questions which come naturally to the lips is more important than following a set of rules. In recent years, the use of validated instruments, such as the HAD (Zigmond and Snaith 1983) and the KGV (Krawiecka et al. 1977), has become common. Nursing staff have embraced them as a useful way of exploring aspects of mental state. As is evident, we are instinctively antagonistic to questionnaires, forms and standardised instruments in clinical practice. Nonetheless, experience has shown that they have a role. Indeed, there are good grounds to think that they can be more effective in eliciting psychopathology than less structured approaches. They cannot, however, replace clinical skills.

BOX 3.1 The General Schema for Recording Mental State Examination

- Appearance
- Behaviour
- Mood
- Speech
- Disorders of the form of thought
- Abnormal beliefs
- Abnormal perceptions
- Other qualitatively abnormal experiences
- Phobic symptoms
- Obsessive-compulsive symptoms
- Ideas of self-harm
- Ideas of harming others
- Cognitive testing
- Insight

Mental state examination is usually recorded following a schema like that shown in Box 3.1. This is not a guide for conducting a mental state examination. Mental state is examined throughout the interview. Psychopathology is explored opportunistically, as it arises naturally, as part of history taking, or in more informal parts of the conversation. Inexperienced and unskilled interviewers often try to conduct mental state examination as a formal exercise. They follow the schema and systematically ask questions about a large range of potential psychopathologies, most of which the patient has not experienced. As trainees in large mental hospitals, we both witnessed such interviews in ward rounds conducted by consultants who seemed to feel a need to emulate Charcot.[1] As trainers we have watched trainees struggling to elicit psychopathology in a similar fashion. Patients experience this, at best, as puzzling and irrelevant, and, at worst, as humiliating and anxiety provoking. It is also ineffective. Furthermore, serial mental state interrogations are an extremely unreliable way of judging the progress of treatment or changes in the patient's mental health.

The best clinical interviewers approach mental state examination in a conversational and informal manner. A conversational approach relaxes the patient, who is then better able to explain their experiences. Questions that relate to the patient's concerns and daily activities are more likely to elicit psychopathologies, because this is the context in which they are experienced.

In general, people suffering from anxiety or depression are readily able to describe psychopathology, as they recognise the nature of symptoms, including that they arise from within themselves. Even when depression is so severe that delusions develop, the anguish associated with the condition means that the patient usually wants to talk about it.

In acute schizophreniform psychosis, patients often attribute experiences that are part of their illness to the activities of others, which can create a problem in getting them to tell you about all of the symptoms that are relevant. In mania, patients may not believe there is any

---

[1] Jean-Martin Charcot was a nineteenth-century Parisian neurologist whose public lectures featured dramatic demonstrations of hypnosis and patients with 'hysterical' symptoms. The young Sigmund Freud attended and was duly impressed.

problem at all. Milder forms of mania can be very difficult to assess in interviews. This is especially true during the recovery phase of the first episode. The patient, lacking previous experience of being unwell, finds it hard to identify remaining symptoms, and may not yet recognise that they have been ill. The clinician has no experience of the patient as a person, and therefore cannot judge whether the improvement represents a return to their normal self or not. Asking decontextualised questions about whether thoughts are still racing, whether they feel they have special abilities, whether they are making ill-judged decisions, and so on, are unlikely to elicit remaining problems. More fruitful is a discussion as to what they have been doing, what concerns they have, what plans they are making and how they are getting on with their family. Although it is still possible to miss residual psychopathology, this focus on the tangible and the relevant is likely to expose the way that the patient is thinking, how they have been behaving and therefore what psychopathology is still present. This general principle applies in a range of situations where psychopathology is hard to elicit.

Deciding what type of psychopathology is present can also be difficult. We have noticed over a long period of time that trainees are reluctant to ask obvious, commonsense questions. This is unfortunate, as these questions more often illuminate psychopathology than do more formal, structured questions. The best questions tend to be 'What?' 'Why?' 'Who?' and 'How?' For example, 'What is it that keeps distracting your attention?' 'Why are you so tense at the moment?' 'How is it possible for people to interfere with your thoughts?' 'Why are the CIA bothering to follow you?' or even simply 'How does that work, then?' If a patient wears sunglasses throughout an interview in an ordinarily lit room, it may be in conformity to fashion, or because they have a black eye, or because they are paranoid or for some other reason. The only way of understanding is to ask why.

Sometimes it is necessary, towards the end of the interview, to ask direct questions about symptoms which may not have been mentioned earlier. What is to be avoided is asking a blitz of stereotyped questions about every potential mental state abnormality. It is possible to get suggestible people to agree that they have every symptom you mention. It is better to use probe questions than menus of potential symptoms, and we give some examples below. To reiterate, above all it is important to help patients to explain what they are actually experiencing rather than browbeating them to give a classical, but inaccurate, account of their symptoms.

On the question of note keeping, it is normally best to write down the exact nature of any mental state abnormality as soon as you have a clear description, as details are often forgotten by the end of even brief interviews. It is no good to record that delusions and hallucinations (or any other psychopathologies) are present without writing down as much as you possibly can about the nature and content of these. You, and others, will need this information at a later time. It is best to record in as much detail as possible, and verbatim examples are especially helpful.

The only way to become skilled at mental state examination is to talk with lots of patients, not just as part of formal clinical interviews, but also informally. There is absolutely no substitute for sitting and talking over a cup of coffee. Clinical interviewing can only offer a certain level of understanding of what it is like to be mentally ill. Knowing patients in more relaxed moments assists in developing a more profound understanding of the nature of mental illness. It helps you to see not just what is wrong, but also what is preserved; to understand the effect of mental illness on ordinary everyday activities; and to witness certain types of experiences as they actually happen, rather than through retrospective accounts.

The strength of nursing is that nurses do this all the time. One of the weaknesses of psychiatrists is that doctors tend to feel that they should remain aloof. Modern patterns of psychiatric work have made it more difficult to chat, but it is not impossible if you understand its value.

Appearance and Behaviour

This is generally the most neglected part of mental state examination, perhaps due to the lack of operationalised categories of abnormality in appearance and behaviour. However, the ability to observe is an absolute prerequisite for doing mental state examination well. Observation is an active process. You have to be able to notice what is there. If appearance and behaviour are unusual, you have to be able to break the observation down into component parts and work out exactly what is not right.

Observation extends beyond spotting outlandish clothing or strange behaviour. Thirty years ago, one of us interviewed a very depressed man who was unable to give much information about himself. In a moment of drifting attention, the psychiatrist noticed that there was a blob at the end of each hair on his head, and correctly surmised that his hair had been burned. When asked how this had happened, the man explained that he saved on paying barbers by burning his hair with a match. The revelation opened up many issues about his long-term functioning and his ability to care for himself.

Mood

Although attempts have been made to define a distinction between 'mood' and 'affect' by reference to cryptic metaphors about climate (mood) and weather (affect), for all practical purposes they mean the same thing. Mood is not a unidimensional emotion on a happiness–sadness continuum, with depression and mania at the extremes and euthymia in the middle. It has a complex, multifaceted quality. Within normal experience, 'happiness' can include contentment, blissfulness, restless excitement and playfulness, each having some unique qualities. Furthermore, mood is reactive to circumstances. It modulates and changes over short periods of time, against a background of more persistent prevailing feelings. The standard psychopathological descriptions set out the major mood abnormalities (depression, elation, anxiety, anger, perplexity). These can coexist in all combinations, including elation and depression (in so-called mixed affective states), and depression and anger. The clinical description of mood involves recognition of these subtleties.

The identification of disorders of reactivity and modulation of mood is difficult. The most straightforward is labile, or abnormally reactive, mood. This is part of the manic syndrome, but it can occur in other circumstances. For example, people who are anxious often shift quickly from nervous giggling to tears.

The converse state, flattened affect (the loss of normal modulation and reactivity of mood) is more troublesome. We normally think of this as the emotional component of the negative symptoms of chronic schizophrenia, where it is associated with a lack of drive and volition, with an apparent indifference to the environment. However, people who are depressed frequently show marked flattening of affect, as their misery prevents them from engaging emotionally with the outside world. Many psychotropic drugs can induce flattened affect, giving rise to the familiar complaint 'This stuff makes me feel like a zombie'. People with disorders on the autistic spectrum may show very little emotional modulation. Some people, otherwise entirely emotionally well, habitually display a dour, emotionless affect, sometimes as a backdrop to a mordant wit. Each of these very different situations can give rise to a similar clinical presentation of flattened affect. Some care is needed to tell them apart.

Incongruous affect presents similar difficulties. Although there may be a variety of types of incongruous affect, in practice it almost always presents as giggling for no evident reason. This is a symptom of acute schizophreniform psychosis. It is especially common in hebephrenic states, which are dominated by thought disorder, perplexity and strange behaviour, sometimes in the absence of consistent and prominent delusions and hallucinations. Hebephrenia commonly occurs in adolescence. Giggling is often a response to remarks made by hallucinatory voices, in which case it is actually a congruous response to an abnormal experience. In addition to this, thought disorder and general disorganisation of mental functioning can make people see humour where others see none, and this is usually apparent when you ask them what is funny. However, every schoolteacher knows that disaffected, awkward teenagers use giggling as a strategy of defiance. Some people try to control anxiety through a sort of humourless flippancy. One of the major behavioural consequences of cannabis intoxication is incongruous giggling.

There is a range of causes of incongruous giggling which are especially common in young people, only some of which are related to mental illness. Asking what is funny (in a curious rather than an affronted or challenging manner) may or may not clarify matters.

Generally speaking, abnormalities of mood are easy to detect through observation and listening throughout an interview. Changes in mood have profound effects on the minutiae of behaviour, and ordinary empathic social interaction involves detecting and responding to the other person's mood. Despite this, it is important to ask people about their mood (e.g. 'What has your mood been like?') because a minority of people hide depression behind a smiling mask, which only slips in response to a direct question about their feelings.

Asking about factors that provoke changes in mood can help distinguish the true diurnal variation of severe depression (worse in the morning, better in the afternoon) from diurnal patterns sustained by other factors, for example the arrival home of a partner. You should also ask about irritability and the typical precipitants for irritable outbursts. These are not always spontaneously mentioned, and they can be important in assessing the atmosphere in the household and behaviour towards family, especially children.

Where depression is present, questions about despair and hopelessness are the most reliable indicators of its severity. Probes are best aimed at establishing what the patient thinks is going to happen to them, for example 'Do you think you're likely to get better eventually?' This then leads naturally to questions about suicidal thoughts, for example 'Has it ever got so bad you've thought of killing yourself?' Assessment of risk is an important subject, and we deal with it in Chapter 19.

We have mentioned alterations in appetite, sleep and concentration in the previous chapter, but in the sequence of an interview, you often ask about them alongside questions about mood.

Thought and Speech

Under this heading you are interested in the *form* rather than the *content* of thought, hence the term 'formal thought disorder', the adjective meaning 'of form' rather than 'proper'. Of course, thought is entirely inaccessible to other people, and it can only be accessed through the intermediary of speech. It is important to be vigilant for speech problems when assessing whether there is formal thought disorder. Thought disorder has a high diagnostic weighting, and schizophreniform thought disorder is sometimes regarded as pathognomonic (i.e. it occurs exclusively in that disorder).

There are a number of speech disorders. The most common are subcultural inarticulacy, stuttering and dysphasia. The first of these is due to lack of self-confidence, often based on poor education, leading to restricted vocabulary and fluency. It displays itself in muddled speech combined with difficulty in elaborating and explaining. This demands patience and encouragement from the interviewer, as it tends to improve when the person is relaxed.

Stuttering is not always obvious when the person has learned to control it. Techniques to control stuttering include pausing, looking for alternative words or altering the direction of what is being said. This can induce an odd quality to the person's speech, which can become hesitant or sometimes a little robotic.

Dysphasia is a frequent sequel of brain injury. It often affects older people after strokes (cerebrovascular accidents), but it is also common in younger people after closed head injuries (e.g. in road traffic accidents), sub-arachnoid haemorrhage and encephalitis. The most common problem is in word finding. As with stuttering, many people find an accommodation to the problem, which can make their speech sound unusual. They stop and try to find a different expression, or repeatedly use the same word to stand in for words they cannot find. Some people use a stock obscenity, as such words are grammatically flexible ('Oh fuck, the fucking fucker's fucking fucked': expletive, adjective, noun, adverb and verb). This makes them seem foul-mouthed and socially disinhibited. Where a less offensive word is used, it can give the impression of using a neologism (see below). The possibility of dysphasia should be borne in mind wherever there is a history of head or brain injury.

In mania and hypomania, the classical descriptions of pressure of speech and flight of ideas do hold true. Everything is speeded up and the person endlessly digresses, their ability to follow a logical thread severely compromised by punning, alliteration, rhyming, clang associations and so forth. Lesser degrees of this (so-called *prolixity*) are hard to assess, as similar over-inclusive, digressive thinking is commonly seen in people who are pedantic by nature. It is also seen in the habitually garrulous. Some people with very obsessional personalities are so concerned with completeness that they have to speak quickly in order to avoid their digressions being interrupted, and this can resemble hypomanic prolixity.

Schizophreniform formal thought disorder is undoubtedly a key feature of the condition, though it is far from invariable. Whilst experience improves most clinical skills, it can be an impediment to the recognition of this type of thought disorder. Psychiatrists come to understand their patients' preoccupations, experiences and lifestyle. When they suffer an acute relapse of psychosis, you can follow their train of thought. Years of familiarity with disordered thinking rob it of the quality of oddness, which ordinarily is the most striking feature. The only way we know of overcoming this is to try and spot the main features as a deliberate exercise. Although you rarely encounter thought disorder that exactly conforms to the classical descriptions, the discipline is helpful in detecting formal abnormalities. Some of the features are set out in Box 3.2.

Abnormal Beliefs

There are a number of definitions of a delusion, which can be summarised as: 'a false and unshakeable belief, which is out of keeping with the patient's social and cultural

> **BOX 3.2** Some Features of Schizophreniform Thought Disorder
>
> - Concrete thinking: a failure of abstract thinking where metaphor takes on a literal quality.
> - Loosening of associations: ideas lack proper links, which gives a 'woolly' and inconclusive quality to what is said.
> - Over-inclusiveness and interpenetration of themes: clarity of thinking is lost because too many ideas are linked together.
> - Logical failures: more severe than simple woolliness, thinking shows 'derailment' or 'knight's move' and, without acknowledgement, the train of thought alters completely. This often is related to the intrusion of a completely unrelated concept.
> - Neologisms: strictly speaking the use of an invented word to describe a phenomenon outside of ordinary experience, but more commonly the use of an existing word in an idiosyncratic and bizarre way (e.g. a patient complained of 'email', meaning thoughts inserted by other people, which he thought was due to the use of ecstasy, i.e. MDMA or 'E').
> - Drivelling: an unfortunate and unpleasant term for a common feature of thought disorder; syntax and grammar are preserved, but thinking becomes so muddled and disorganised that the person appears to be talking for no reason, and conveys nothing.
> - Word-salad: the total breakdown of all syntactical and grammatical structure where thinking becomes a series of unrelated words.

background'. Delusions are the most common symptom of psychosis and they generally conform to this conventional definition. The definition is, however, inadequate. Every element is subject to major exceptions (delusions can be true, they are not necessarily totally unshakeable, and other people who are not mentally ill may share similar beliefs). Furthermore, some beliefs (for example, some spiritual, religious and political ideas adhered to with fanatical intensity) meet the criteria without being conventionally regarded as delusional. The use of the concept of the 'over-valued idea', which is applied to delusion-like ideas, only adds to the confusion.

For example, people with anorexia nervosa often believe that they are fat, when objectively they are thin. This is said to be an over-valued idea, but the only reason for regarding it as anything other than a delusion is convenience. It is regarded as unhelpful and misleading to conceptualise anorexia nervosa as a psychosis. There are quite a few other problems and overlaps in addition to these, for example the over-expansive ideas and plans of the grandiose wishful thinker, whose expectations are not strictly impossible but are extremely unlikely to come to fruition.

It would be nice to think that someone will produce an evidence-based approach to sort these problems out, but for now we just have to accept that there are ambiguities, and that from time to time you are bound to come across situations where it is hard to tell if someone is deluded or not. The most useful question in making the assessment is 'How do you know that?' Exploration of the logic behind a strange belief usually gives you some sense as to whether it is delusional or not.

Delusions are said to be either primary or secondary. Primary delusions come with a quality of sudden insight, or even epiphany ('I suddenly knew what was happening') and are said to be unrelated to other ideas or evidence. Primary delusions are almost always preceded by a delusional mood, a strong sense that something indefinable is wrong with the world, neatly but unwittingly captured by Bob Dylan in the lyric *Something is happening here but you don't know what it is, do you, Mister Jones?'* The formation of the delusion carries a crystallising sense of understanding.

Kurt Schneider, delineating his first rank symptoms (Schneider 1959), referred to delusional perceptions rather than primary delusions. A delusional perception is a sudden delusional belief linked to an unrelated perception ('The television flickered and I realised my father was Satan'). In our experience, it is difficult to find these phenomena unless you interview the patient very early in the development of the illness. This may be because these specific phenomena become lost amongst explanatory elaborations and other secondary symptoms.

It is always important to fully explore delusional ideas. Delusions about specific individuals in the immediate environment are quite likely to lead the person to take some form of action and this may involve risk to all concerned. For example, men with jealous delusions about their partners often make accusations and some go on to act aggressively. It is always important to ask people what they intend to do about delusional beliefs. Even where delusions are held about remote figures or appear relatively benign, people can get into terrible trouble through acting upon them, for example by trying to contact famous people under delusions of mutual love.

When people have acute psychosis, delusional beliefs are highly salient, which is to say they loom large in their awareness, and they are usually very bothered by them. Under these circumstances, delusions are not difficult to elicit. When psychosis is controlled by medication, or where the person has been continuously unwell for years, the ideas often persist but salience diminishes. They come to resemble unusual opinions, and they may not be mentioned spontaneously. Some people, deluded and preoccupied, nonetheless recognise that their ideas sound peculiar, or come to realise that professionals regard them as evidence of mental disorder. All of these situations can make delusions hard to elicit. There are no general-purpose probes that will reliably lead to disclosure of delusions under these circumstances. You have to probe about specific ideas that the individual has expressed in the past, or which an informant mentions as an odd idea that the person has expressed. In other words, you are dependent on personal or second-hand prior knowledge of the patient. In the UK this is universally referred to (somewhat disrespectfully) as 'knowing what buttons to press'. Once the relevant ideas have been raised, even the most guarded person with delusions will talk about them.

Abnormal Perceptions

Auditory Hallucinations

By far the most common abnormal perceptions are 'voices'. They were once believed to mainly affect people with schizophrenia and organic cerebral lesions, but it is now clear that significant numbers of people with neither diagnosis experience them (Van Os et al. 2000; Daalman et al. 2011). At present, there is no exhaustive classification of 'voices'. For example, people with borderline personality disorder often complain of hearing voices. They are often thought to be either describing unpleasant thoughts or else just making it up. However, their complaints of voices are consistent, and it is a very poor principle to assume that groups of patients lie about their experiences. Modern functional imaging studies show similar patterns of brain activation when complaining of voices in people with schizophrenia and personality disorder.

A wide range of organic factors can induce hallucinations, some specific, such as high doses of amphetamine-like drugs, and some non-specific, such as delirium. Some types of hallucination are clearly organic in origin, but the mechanisms by which they are induced are obscure. A prominent example is alcoholic hallucinosis, which occurs after years of heavy drinking, and can persist through months of abstinence. The hallucinosis is mainly auditory, and arises without fixed delusions or other psychotic phenomena.

Organic hallucinations generally have a vivid, concrete and frightening quality. Where there is no clouding of consciousness, the false perceptions have the same quality as true perceptions. However, the person can readily pick up on environmental clues that they are 'hearing things'. People suffering from organic hallucinosis are particularly likely to show major behavioural responses to hallucinations. Where the person vigorously converses with hallucinations, you should always suspect an organic origin. The features of organic hallucinosis are evident in solitary heavy drinkers, who can be seen in city centres throughout the Western world. They shout aggressively, but when approached they are usually entirely pleasant. They will freely acknowledge that they are shouting at voices, not because they think they are real, but because shouting makes them feel better. They will volunteer that their heavy alcohol consumption causes the voices.

Conversely, whilst people with schizophrenia are usually certain that auditory hallucinations are real, it is clear that they have a very different quality to true perceptions. The vast majority of people who suffer schizophreniform auditory hallucinations, when asked whether they hear voices, confirm that they do. Although they believe that the voices are authentic perceptions, they recognise a different quality to other perceptions. Although the classical auditory hallucinations of schizophrenia are in the third person, second-person auditory hallucinations are equally common.

Behavioural responses to hallucinations in schizophrenia tend to be limited to pausing and listening or looking at the places where voices seem to be coming from, though active replying to voices does occur. This is most frequently a sub-vocal muttering.

Traditionally, the distinction between hallucinations and non-hallucinatory 'voices' turns upon whether the experience arises within subjective or objective space. This has led to the widespread practice of asking people whether the voices arise from within their head or not. In our opinion, the use of this question is to be avoided, as it does not clarify the nature of the experience. The distinction really turns upon whether the false perception is experienced as arising from within the self or elsewhere. The self has no anatomical or geometric location. The crucial question to ask is: what does the patient think causes the voices? If the cause is entirely external, then the experience is more likely to be a hallucination, though this is not absolute, as some people have partially self, partially non-self explanations for hallucinations.

The content of hallucinations should be explored if you can, although many people with voices find it hard clearly to describe what they hear. Fragmentary, derogatory hallucinations can occur in severe depression, but they are more common in schizophrenia. The diagnostic value of exploring content is not great, but it is important in understanding what the patient is experiencing.

Command hallucinations are significant. These are hallucinations that instruct the person what to do. Simply asking 'Do the voices ever tell you what to do?' is usually sufficient to elicit them. Command hallucinations are relatively common. A minority of patients follow the hallucinatory instructions, often after long periods of resistance. This can create serious risks. Where there are command hallucinations, you need fully to explore the content and the factors, if any, which restrain the person from acting upon them.

Non-Auditory Hallucinations

Hallucinations can, of course, arise in any sensory modality, and sometimes completely outside of the usual sensorium (for example, powerful feelings of an invisible presence). Non-auditory hallucinations in psychosis are frequently ambiguous experiences, somewhere between hallucinations, delusions and delusional misinterpretations of normal experiences, for example the feeling of worms crawling under the skin, or of something alive in the abdomen. Visual hallucinations are more common in schizophrenia than traditional teaching suggested (Cutting 1990), and these are sometimes associated with complex multi-modality experiences (for example, demonic shadows that enter the bedroom, whose hot breath can be heard and felt against the skin).

Pseudo-Hallucinations and Related Phenomena

There are several psychopathologies that are broadly similar to true hallucinations. It can be very hard to distinguish delusions of reference from hallucinations. According to the classical descriptions, delusions of reference are beliefs that neutral and impersonal materials, such as television programmes or car number plates, carry a personal and intentional message. However, patients often report that the television or other media do not allude to them but actually mention them by name or show pictures of them. The difference can be significant in distinguishing persistent delusional disorder (where there are delusions but no auditory hallucinations or other psychotic phenomena) from schizophrenia (which is more likely to respond well to treatment). Obsessional ruminations are sometimes first mentioned as 'voices', because of their repetitive and unwelcome quality. As stated earlier, some people describe experiences intermediate between ruminations and delusions and/or hallucinations.

The most vexed issue is that of pseudo-hallucinations. There are a number of different definitions, and the term is a semantic nonsense, meaning 'false false perception'. In practice, the term is applied to a wide variety of experiences, and it is common for the semantic confusion to be replicated by mental health professionals in statements such as 'she's been complaining of hearing voices, but we don't think they're real voices'. *None* of the experiences that we refer to as 'voices' are objectively real. The sub-text is usually that the patient is complaining of a psychotic symptom without any other sign of psychosis, and is therefore disbelieved. It is, however, dangerous to leap to the conclusion that people are feigning psychotic symptoms. As a rule of thumb (based on experience), when you are 100 per cent certain that a patient is feigning psychotic symptoms, there is a 50 per cent chance that, in the fullness of time, they will turn out to have been mentally ill all along.

In practice, the only way that we have been able to resolve the issue of pseudo-hallucinations has been to accept that there is a heterogeneous group of experiences that are very similar to hallucinations. These either occur in the absence of any other evidence of psychosis or cerebral disorder, or they arise with a simultaneous awareness that, whilst they sound 'real', they are not.

Pseudo-hallucinations in the absence of psychosis are often associated with emotional distress. The distress seems to be the cause of, rather than a consequence of, the pseudo-hallucinations. There are two major exceptions. The first is Charles Bonnet syndrome.

This is common. It arises in older people when they develop a visual impairment. They have single modality visual experiences, mostly complex and vivid and often involving tiny people or animals, but sometimes more rudimentary than this. The experiences may lead to distress, which is relieved when the cause is explained. The second exception is a small group of individuals in the general population, neither evidently mentally disordered nor distressed, who have a strong religious faith and who hear the voice of God in their everyday lives. We recognise that they may be right about the origin of the experience, but we prefer to believe that it is due to some other, as yet poorly understood, psychological process.

Flashbacks

In the 1985 edition of Fish's book, the word 'flashback' does not even appear in the index; it appeared for the first time in the 2007 edition (Casey and Kelly 2007). Between the two editions, these experiences attracted an enormous amount of attention. The term was originally used to describe the return of symptoms of intoxication with hallucinogenic drugs (mainly LSD) long after discontinuation. However, the term is now commonly used with respect to vivid and intrusive mental images of distressing experiences. Flashbacks are usually triggered by a trivial reminder of the past experience (a smell or a sound, for example). Although they are transient, they can be intensely upsetting. They were first described in post-traumatic stress disorder (PTSD), and were initially regarded as the most characteristic feature of the syndrome. The fact that they have proven to be common in adult survivors of childhood sexual abuse has led some researchers to the view that the adult consequences of abuse are a form of PTSD (e.g. Ackerman et al. 1998). However, such experiences seem to be common in the whole population. They can relate to memories that are upsetting or even just embarrassing, and we do not believe that they can be regarded as intrinsically pathological at all. The degree of emotional distress they provoke is more relevant than whether they are present or not.

There are now consistent findings that adults who have been abused as children are more likely to experience hallucinations and other psychotic symptoms (with or without psychosis per se) (Shevlin et al. 2007, Bentall et al. 2012). There may be relatively specific associations between the type of abuse and the modality of hallucinations. Tactile hallucinations, for example, appear to be more common amongst people who have been physically (rather than emotionally) abused. These findings create an ambiguity over the distinction between flashbacks and hallucinations. It has no resolution at present. This underlines the importance of being clear about exactly what patients are describing when they complain of 'flashbacks'.

Other Psychotic Symptoms

There are many other symptoms that can arise in psychosis, but the most important, and most common, are passivity experiences and disorders of the possession of thought. These are Schneiderian first rank symptoms of schizophrenia, and they carry some diagnostic significance.

The subjective quality of passivity experiences is that thoughts, actions or (rarely) emotions are literally under the control of an external agency. This is not a conclusion that the person arrives at; it is something they experience. There is usually a technological rationalisation (that this is achieved through computers or satellites), although sometimes

> **BOX 3.3** A Cautionary Tale
>
> A 35-year-old man was admitted to hospital after an unexplained and serious attempt on his own life. In the course of a six-week admission, the only abnormality that he displayed was episodes of 'going blank' and staring at walls. These episodes happened several times a day. In interviews with the psychiatrist, he could explain neither the suicide attempt nor the 'blank' episodes. Eventually, the clinical team came to the conclusion that the presentation could be convincingly understood in terms of a dissociative state. The psychiatrist carefully explained the idea to the patient, who enthusiastically agreed that this made a lot of sense. It was decided he should go home, and he went off to make the necessary arrangements. Realising that they had not discussed plans for further treatment, the psychiatrist asked the nurses what the patient was doing, and was told he was busy phoning his father.
>
> Eventually, the patient returned, and the psychiatrist said 'You've been phoning your father.' The patient asked how he knew this, and the psychiatrist, in a moment of inappropriate flippancy, said 'Telepathy'. The patient simply nodded. The psychiatrist found this odd, so he said 'That was a joke.' The patient replied 'Well, there's a lot of it going on!' The patient had catatonic schizophrenia. The psychiatrist was one of us.

the supernatural is blamed (demons, Satan or witchcraft). These experiences are usually volunteered as you explore delusional beliefs. The probe 'Do you ever feel that someone else is controlling what you think?' tends not to be very helpful, as a large number of people feel that a parent, their partner or authority in general is excessively controlling. Hence a lot of people say yes. It can be confusing to try to disentangle the effect of everyday resentment towards an over-controlling relative from true passivity experiences. Even asking 'How do they do that?' may not clarify matters. The probe 'Does anyone interfere with your thinking?' tends to work better, and will tend to elicit disorders of the possession of thought as well as passivity experiences.

The disorders of the possession of thought include hearing your own thoughts spoken out loud, thought insertion, thought withdrawal, and thought broadcasting. Although the term 'thought broadcasting' suggests that the person feels that everyone can hear their thoughts, it more commonly involves one or more specific individuals who can hear them. Like passivity experiences, this is usually rationalised in technological terms, such as the presence of implanted brain probes. There is potential confusion with an everyday experience here too, as most of us have people in our lives who can 'read' us or can 'tell what we're thinking'. Traditional probes such as 'Are your thoughts private?' or 'Are your thoughts your own?' seem to convey little meaning even to people who are experiencing thought broadcasting. The more direct question 'Do you ever feel there's telepathy going on?' seems to work better (Box 3.3).

Anxiety Symptoms

Anxiety symptoms are rarely difficult to elicit. They are likely to be volunteered early in the interview. Where they are not, there is no reason to avoid asking, 'Do you have any phobias?' and 'Have you ever had a panic attack?' as these words are part of the general vocabulary, and if the person does not understand, it is easy to explain. However, people sometimes use the terms in idiosyncratic ways, so it is important to clarify what they mean.

Phobias are, of course, incredibly common and come in an enormous variety of forms and degrees of severity. Psychiatrists regularly encounter unusual phobias, such as the fear of buttons or the fear of moderately severe injury. Some people have an unusual variant of social phobia where they can cope with good friends and complete strangers, but are anxious around people they know slightly. They fail to attend the second interview.

Phobias have two essential features: fear of a situation or thing, and avoidance. Avoidance can, however, take a number of different forms. Many people with agoraphobia go out and about when accompanied (which is avoidance of being alone in the feared situation), and many people with social phobia cope with social situations by getting very intoxicated with alcohol or cannabis, which is a type of chemically mediated avoidance.

Panic attacks are extremely unpleasant but short-lived (though some people experience serial panic attacks). Where people report that the experience has lasted 20 minutes or more, it is unlikely to have been a panic attack (although people can overestimate the duration because it is so distressing). They are characterised by a feeling of terror, a sense of imminent death or catastrophe, and an overwhelming desire to flee. Usually there are strong physiological concomitants such as palpitations and sweating. The majority of sufferers feel short of breath during an attack, and this is due to hyperventilation. A minority of people with panic attacks do not hyperventilate.

Anxiety symptoms in people with severe depression or schizophreniform psychosis tend to be neglected by assessing clinicians as they are regarded as secondary to the underlying problem. Patients are always bothered by anxiety. It is hard to bear and it deserves to be properly explored. It is important to appreciate that anxiety can be a significant risk factor for suicide. This is counter-intuitive. If anxiety is the fear that something bad is about to happen, it seems to makes no sense to deliberately make something bad happen. When people are very anxious in the context of feeling paranoid or depressed, they may see no hope and attempt suicide simply to stop feeling as they do. Risk assessment is discussed in Chapter 19.

Obsessions and Compulsions

We have already discussed the overlap between obsessional symptoms and psychotic symptoms. Obsessional phenomena are extremely common and some people develop such symptoms when they are depressed or when they become anxious about a situational problem. People are often embarrassed by these symptoms, because they tend to focus on themes of contamination, violence and sexuality, so that it is often necessary to ask about them specifically. Probes about the tendency to check things excessively (for example, doors and windows at night or the gas before going out) usually work. In general, checking accompanies all other obsessional symptoms. Even when people deny checking, they usually understand the point of the question and reveal other obsessional symptoms if they are present.

Obsessional thoughts are repetitive and distressing. The term 'obsessional rumination' is a rare example of the use of a poetically evocative term in psychiatry. Rumination comes from the Latin verb *ruminare*, which means to chew the cud as cows do. Obsessional thoughts are ego dystonic (i.e. contrary to the person's wishes or values), but are unequivocally perceived as arising from within the self. They are experienced as senseless. Initially they are resisted, although resistance leads to rising anxiety. Compulsions are behaviours aimed at controlling obsessions, and involve ritualised activity, often centred on cleaning or counting. In severe obsessive-compulsive disorder (OCD), there is usually marked avoidance, and there can be bizarre manoeuvres to achieve this, such as wrapping oneself in plastic to avoid contamination or chaining oneself to the bed to avoid a nocturnal act of violence. It has long been recognised, however, that no single feature is invariable. This can make it very difficult to distinguish obsessional phenomena from other types of symptoms.

There are two non-psychotic phenomena which are similar to obsessions, but which are more likely to be acted upon. The first is the resisted intention. Here, the person wants to do something, usually an act of violence, but resists because of the consequences. An example would be the father of a rape victim who feels fully justified in seriously assaulting the perpetrator, but is begged by his family to do nothing for fear of the consequences. He is utterly preoccupied by thoughts of violence. They are resisted and they are accompanied by severe emotional turmoil. Vengeful resisted intentions may be provoked by less understandable affronts. For example, they may be directed at blameless hospital staff who have attended the death of a loved one, or the perpetrator of a perceived social snubbing. Similar resisted intentions are seen in some people who are struggling with personality-based difficulties with aggression or sexuality during the build-up to a serious offence.

The second type of phenomenon is compulsion-like urges. These closely correspond to the non-psychiatric usage of the word 'compulsion'. The person has a rising sense of psychological tension and feels increasingly compelled to carry out a particular act. There is resistance, but eventually the act is carried out. This initially leads to a profound sense of relief, but this in turn is often followed by feelings of self-disgust or fear of discovery. These experiences arise in a range of problems with very different origins, including bulimia, repeated self-laceration, some types of sexual exhibitionism ('flashing') and substance misuse.

Ideas of Self-Harm and of Harming Others

Needless to say, patients should be asked about thoughts of harming themselves or somebody else. If these are present they must be fully explored, including those factors that restrain them from action. Risk assessment is dealt with in more detail in Chapter 19.

Insight

The idea that there is a continuum of insight from full to none, and that insight can be quantified, is simply wrong. Unqualified terms like 'no insight' and 'good insight' have very little meaning, other than in indicating the extent to which the patient agrees with the psychiatrist as to what is wrong with them. As psychiatrists can be mistaken, this conveys some information about the relationship, but very little about the patient. What is more relevant is how the patient understands their situation and what they think is likely to be helpful. For example, many people with psychotic illnesses believe their delusions to be true, but readily accept efforts to help them. They often have a sophisticated understanding of how the balance of stress and medication alters the severity of symptoms. Whether this is good or poor insight is irrelevant (one could argue the case either way), but an understanding of their attitude has real practical importance. It would be more appropriate to label this section as 'patient's understanding of the problem', which implies something more nuanced than 'insight'.

Main Points in This Chapter

1. Mental state examination rests upon careful observation and listening.
2. There are some real ambiguities regarding psychopathology, but the traditional framework is a helpful guide, provided one recognises its limitations.
3. Probe questions about psychopathology are best framed with reference to activities and ideas that are familiar to the patient. Abstract, 'technical' questions do not work very well.
4. It is important to avoid the trap whereby prior assumptions about the nature of the problem lead to a misinterpretation of what you are told.
5. Even experienced, skilled interviewers sometimes miss important psychopathology.

Cognitive State Examination and Organic Disease

No matter what you believe with regard to the general usefulness of the 'medical model' in mental health, there is one excellent reason for the close involvement of doctors in the care of people with mental disorders. The full range of psychiatric disorders can be mimicked by physical disease. There are no exceptions. The effects of physical illness, and of the drugs that are used to treat it, frequently complicate mental illness. People with chronic mental health problems suffer from more physical ill health than the rest of the population (Hert et al. 2011). Psychiatrists draw upon their background knowledge of physical medicine far more frequently than is commonly appreciated by the rest of the medical profession. *Lishman's Organic Psychiatry* (David et al. 2009), now in its fourth edition as a multi-author text, is an essential purchase for all clinical psychiatrists. The earlier editions (e.g. Lishman 1997) are a little out of date, but they are outstanding works of single-author scholarship. They are beautifully well written and they are worth reading for this reason alone.

Some sub-specialties, such as old-age psychiatry and neuropsychiatry, are primarily concerned with the psychological effects of physical disease. Organic factors commonly cause concern in all forms of psychiatric practice, including child psychiatry and psychotherapy. All mental health practitioners must have the ability to recognise the possibility that physical disorder may be contributing to a problem. Whilst this may mean asking somebody else to evaluate fully the physical or cognitive state, the ability to carry out competently a basic cognitive state assessment is an essential skill for everyone involved in psychiatric practice. Frank cognitive impairment may not be present, or may not be detectable, in all situations where physical disorder is causing psychiatric symptoms. The key to detecting organic pathology is good history taking and careful observation. Cognitive function testing usually serves to confirm or refute the prior impression that there is a cognitive deficit.

There are two major traps as far as organic disorder is concerned. The first is to accept too easily that another doctor has 'excluded' physical disease. Physical disease can rarely be definitively excluded, and an initial belief that a problem is 'psychiatric' can lead doctors into hasty judgements (see Box 4.1).

The second trap is where you have looked for, and failed to find, organic disorder, but it develops (or becomes detectable) later (see Box 4.2). There is a never-to-be-forgotten rule in psychiatry: *the possibility of undisclosed physical disease is part of every differential diagnosis at every stage of treatment.*

The range of interactions between physical disease and psychiatric symptoms is very wide, but the commonest are delirium and dementia.

BOX 4.1 Neurologists Can Be Wrong

A 48-year-old woman with a past history of depression had a first episode of mania. After discharge from hospital she dropped out of follow-up, but was treated by her GP with chlorpromazine 50 mg at night. After two years, she developed writhing, athetoid movements in her right arm and neck. She was sent to see a neurologist, who gave the opinion that this was due to tardive dyskinesia. He advised discontinuation of chlorpromazine. Three weeks later she was seen by a psychiatrist, having developed a relapse of hypomania. The psychiatrist doubted the diagnosis of tardive dyskinesia, which is rarely restricted to one limb. She asked the patient how the symptoms had started. The abnormal movements had commenced in the fingers and over a few weeks spread up the whole arm to the neck. The psychiatrist feared that there was a rapidly expanding space occupying lesion in the patient's basal ganglia, and immediately arranged investigations. MRI scanning showed multiple inflammatory lesions throughout the patient's brain, concentrated in the basal ganglia, and a diagnosis of systemic lupus erythematosus (SLE) was made. SLE probably accounted for both the mood disorder and the abnormal movements. Management proved complex, as steroids worsened the mood disorder and antipsychotics worsened the abnormal movements.

BOX 4.2 Psychiatrists Can Also Be Wrong

A 56-year-old man with hypertension and mild diabetes was referred with a 12-month history of depression. Full assessment, including cognitive testing and a limited range of blood tests, showed no organic explanation and he was treated unsuccessfully with antidepressants. After a series of outpatient attendances over a year, the psychiatrist suddenly noticed that the patient was overweight, with coarse dry hair and a gruff voice. He did everything rather ponderously. Thyroid function tests showed that the results had changed from bottom of the normal range to severely hypothyroid over 12 months. The patient made an excellent recovery on thyroxin, and was remarkably forgiving of the psychiatrist, given that they both came to recognise that the clinical features of myxoedema had been present from the outset.

Delirium

Delirium (sometimes known as 'acute confusional state') is a very common acute event. There is a qualitative alteration in consciousness, with impairment of awareness of the environment. There are specific changes in cognitive processes.

Attention can be neither sustained nor shifted in the normal way. Frequently there are perceptual disturbances, accompanied by disorientation and memory impairment. The experience is subjectively unpleasant and frightening. The person seems to be living through a series of experiences that have a 'bad dream' quality. On recovery, their recollection of the experience is incomplete. The actual clinical presentation can vary widely and all degrees of delirium are seen, from mild and subtle to severe and obvious. No feature is invariable but agitation, hallucinations and paranoid fears are common. As a consequence, delirium can resemble psychosis.

Psychiatrists working in acute hospital liaison services are frequently asked to see delirious patients in medical and surgical wards who are said to have 'gone psychotic'. Box 4.3 sets out a range of causes of delirium.

BOX 4.3 Main Causes of Delirium

- Non-cerebral infections (e.g. lungs, septicaemia)
- Cerebral infections (e.g. meningitis, encephalitis)
- Metabolic problems (e.g. electrolyte disturbance, liver failure, hypoglycaemia)
- Drugs (e.g. intoxication or withdrawal states – especially alcohol)
- Focal brain lesions (e.g. tumour, cerebrovascular lesions, sub-arachnoid and sub-dural haemorrhage)
- Diffuse cerebral problems (e.g. cerebral hypoxia, raised intracranial pressure, multiple inflammatory lesions)
- Head injury
- Nutritional problems (e.g. thiamine deficiency leading to Wernicke's encephalopathy)
- Epilepsy (e.g. post-ictal confusion)

BOX 4.4 Delirium May Not Be Obvious

A 67-year-old widow with chronic obstructive airways disease was assessed by a liaison mental health nurse in the local emergency department. There was a three-day history of schizophreniform symptoms. She complained that her neighbours had been talking about her loudly, accusing her of being a prostitute, and that they had been pumping a poisonous gas through the wall, which she could smell. At night she had been frightened by sensations in her vagina, which she believed were caused by the neighbours having sex with her from next door. She complained that they had been making the patterns on her carpet swirl around in the evenings. She had been making repeated calls to the police about her neighbours, and it was the police who had taken her to hospital. Her concentration was impaired, but there were no other abnormalities on cognitive function testing. On physical examination, she was short of breath and there was evidence of chronic lung disease, but no acute changes were evident. The clinical picture appeared to be typical of late onset paranoid schizophrenia (paraphrenia).

The nurse discussed the patient with the liaison team psychiatrist. On the basis of the short history and the presence of visual perceptual abnormalities in the form of swirling carpet patterns, the psychiatrist wondered about delirium. She suggested that the patient should be given oxygen prior to any decision on treatment. Oxygen abolished all of the psychotic symptoms almost immediately. The patient was admitted to a medical ward, and the next day she showed obvious signs of an acute chest infection. In retrospect, it was clear that this had been developing for several days. On top of existing lung disease, it had been sufficient to cause hypoxia and delirium.

A key feature of delirium is that the severity of the disturbance fluctuates through the 24-hour period. There may be periods of complete or relative lucidity. The disturbance tends to be worse at night, probably because environmental cues for orientation are more ambiguous by night than by day. Other circumstances that make orientation more difficult, such as poor lighting or being left alone, also tend to worsen delirium. Vivid visual hallucinations and visual misperceptions are particularly common. Delirium is not necessarily obvious, but there may be clues from the history or mental state examination (Box 4.4).

BOX 4.5 Main Clinical Features of Delirium

- *Fluctuation* in severity through 24-hour cycle
- *Clouding of consciousness*/inability to direct, focus, sustain or shift attention
- *Disorientation*, especially distorted perception of passage of time
- *Impairment of abstract thinking* and comprehension, including transient delusions
- *Impairment of immediate recall* and of short-term memory
- *Illusions/hallucinations*, especially visual
- *Dysphasia/dysarthria*
- *Psychomotor disturbance*, including hypo- or hyperactivity and enhanced startle reaction
- *Sleep disturbance*, including nightmares with a marked behavioural reaction on waking
- *Emotional disturbance*, including fear, irritability, euphoria, apathy and perplexity

---

BOX 4.6 Dementias/Neurocognitive Disorders

- Neuro-degenerative diseases (e.g. Alzheimer's, Lewy body and Huntington's diseases, fronto-temporal dementia)
- Cerebrovascular (e.g. multi-infarct, cranial arteritis)
- Toxic (e.g. alcohol, heavy metals)
- Nutritional (e.g. thiamine or B12 deficiency)
- Infections (e.g. HIV, Creutzfeldt-Jakob disease, syphilis)
- Structural (e.g. space-occupying lesions, diffuse brain damage such as punch drunk syndrome)
- Anoxia (e.g. after cardiac or respiratory arrest)

A number of conceptual issues concerning delirium have arisen, particularly with regard to the nature of clouding of consciousness and whether a disorder of attention underlies many of the other features. DSM-5 has rather different criteria to DSM-IV for this reason. Nonetheless, delirium has a number of characteristic features that are clinically evident. They are set out in Box 4.5

Dementia/Neurocognitive Disorder

Dementia is a generalised loss of cognitive abilities without disturbance of consciousness. There is a change in intellect, memory and personality. It is caused by a variety of coarse brain diseases, most (though not all) of which are progressive and irreversible. The most common causes of dementia are Alzheimer's disease, cerebrovascular disease (multi-infarct dementia) and Lewy body disease. There are many other causes, some of which are set out in Box 4.6.

Although dementia due to specific diseases may show characteristic symptom patterns and courses, the different disease processes are often difficult to distinguish clinically. All psychiatrists should be able to assess whether dementia is present. Making a reliable definitive diagnosis, on the other hand, is a specialist skill. The degree of impairment on cognitive testing does not necessarily correlate closely to the degree of functional impairment. There may be considerable variation in the degree of cognitive impairment from day to day or hour to hour.

What is Cognitive Testing For?

Clinical cognitive testing is an attempt to make an objective assessment of some cognitive functions during an ordinary clinical interview. It is a much briefer, and less reliable, process than full neuropsychiatric assessment or formal neuropsychological testing. It would be impractical (and not necessarily desirable) to carry out exhaustive testing as a matter of routine clinical practice.

Cognitive function testing is not a good screening tool, as it generates both false positives and false negatives. Generally speaking, if there is nothing in the history to suggest an organic problem, and if mental state examination has not raised a suspicion, then it is very unlikely that cognitive function testing will add anything to the assessment of the case. In reality, few experienced clinicians carry out routine cognitive testing unless there is a reason to do so. However, there is a strong training dictum that it should always be done. To suggest that it should be omitted in professional examinations invites failure. Furthermore, you can only become comfortable with the process, and learn the limits of 'normal', through practice. Whilst you are a trainee, it should be a routine part of a full assessment. If there is a hint of an organic problem, cognitive function testing should always be carried out.

Doing Cognitive Testing

The first thing to say about people with cognitive deficits is that they do not like to be patronised any more than anyone else does. There is no reason why an old and forgetful person should fail to notice that they are being treated discourteously. People who are worried about their cognitive abilities are sensitive to being treated as 'senile'. The relationship between doctor and patient is just as important where the patient has a cognitive deficit as in any other situation. It may be necessary to proceed more slowly, with more explanation and more repetition, but as far as possible people who are cognitively impaired should be treated in the same way as anybody else.

Secondly, just as mental illnesses can be mimicked by organic disease, so all types of cognitive problems can be mimicked by functional mental illness and drug side effects. Interpretation of apparent deficits on cognitive function testing should be made cautiously where the patient is very psychotic, very depressed or very anxious. Unless it is essential to assess cognitive function immediately, it may be best to postpone testing.

Impairment of consciousness should be assessed prior to other testing. If a patient is suffering from significant impairment of consciousness, it can be misleading to comprehensively assess cognitive function, as it is bound to be poor. However, some dementias, such as Lewy body disease, characteristically cause a good deal of fluctuation in cognitive impairment over time. The extent of testing should be adjusted from patient to patient, and should be determined by the clinical question that you are trying to answer. Assessment of delirium in pneumonia is a different process to assessment of Alzheimer's disease.

Box 4.7 sets out the component parts of full consciousness. Any of these may be impaired in normal consciousness, but together the constellation implies general impairment (or clouding) of consciousness. Assessing these rests on observation and clinical judgement. Of these, only attention is amenable to formal testing (using tests of concentration).

> **BOX 4.7** Components of Consciousness (Five As)
>
> - **Awareness**: grasp, knowledge of what is going on in the environment.
> - **Alertness**: readiness to respond, reactivity to stimuli.
> - **Arousal**: overall physiological level of mental activity.
> - **Attention**: the ability to focus on tasks. The ability to sustain attention is concentration.
> - **Awakefulness**: the converse of drowsiness

Standardised Procedures for Cognitive State Assessment

The mini-mental state examination (MMSE) (Anthony et al. 1982) is a validated, internationally recognised clinical screening tool for cognitive impairment. It generates a score that has some clinical relevance when combined with history and other aspects of mental state examination. It can be criticised for being crude and non-specific, and the score it generates is only indicative. It offers a short battery of usable tests that are suitable for everyday purposes. These can be easily memorised, and it is sufficiently robust to suffice as a cognitive state examination in most practical situations, particularly if positive findings can be followed up with more in-depth tests. The MMSE is the only part of this book that we seriously suggest might usefully be learned by rote (Box 4.8).

The MMSE has been in use across the world for decades. It has been subject to a copyright dispute, and efforts have been made to charge for reproduction of scoring sheets with the MMSE printed on them. This has caused some outrage, as clinical procedures are not normally regarded as intellectual property. There is no better procedure for use by non-specialists, and we continue to recommend the items set out in MMSE, which were in use long before MMSE was published.

There are psychometric approaches that are useful in the hands of specialist old age and neuropsychiatrists. However, following a number of reviews (e.g. Lonie et al. 2009) and our own clinical experience, we cannot recommend psychometric procedures in psychiatric practice. They add nothing to ordinary clinical testing.

Further Clinical Cognitive Tests

Most psychiatrists develop a small battery of clinical tests that they use to test specific cognitive functions. These can be used to supplement the items set out in MMSE. It is generally best to develop a relatively small number of tests that you use regularly, as this allows a clearer understanding of the range of normal and abnormal responses. The following is not a comprehensive range of neuropsychiatric tests, but, taken with MMSE items, there is sufficient here for the generalist to make an initial appraisal of cognitive impairment.

Cerebral Dominance

This can be important in localising lesions. Cerebral dominance usually corresponds to handedness, but unfortunately, not always. Footedness and dominant eye can assist in assessing cerebral dominance.

BOX 4.8 Mini-Mental State Examination		
Add points for each correct response		**Points**
Orientation		
1. What is the?	Year?	1
	Season?	1
	Date?	1
	Month?	1
2. Where are we?	State?	1
	Country?	1
	Town?	1
	Hospital?	1
	Floor?	1
Registration		
3. Name three objects, taking one second to say each. Then ask patient to repeat all three. One point for each correct answer. Then repeat the answers until patient learns all three.		3
Attention and calculation		
4. Serial sevens. One point for each correct answer up to five. Alternatively, spell WORLD backwards.		5
Recall		
5. Ask for names of three objects learned in Q.3. One point for each correct answer.		3
Language		
6. Point to a pencil and a watch. Have the patient name them.		2
7. Have the patient repeat 'No ifs, ands or buts'.		1
8. Have the patient follow a three-stage command: 'Take the paper in your right hand. Fold the paper in half. Place the paper on the floor'. One point for each element completed.		3
9. Write in large letters 'CLOSE YOUR EYES'		1
Ask the patient to read and obey.		
10. Have the patient write a sentence of his or her choice. Ignore spelling errors, but it should have a subject and an object, and make sense.		1
Visio-spatial		
11. Enlarge the design below to 1.5 cm per side, and have the patient copy it (give one point if all sides and angles are preserved and if the intersecting sides form a quadrangle).		1

Add points for each correct response	Points
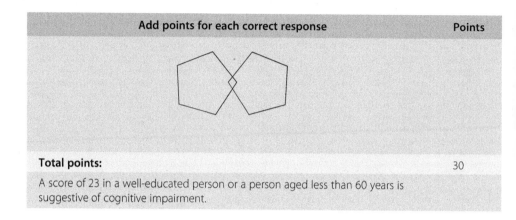	
Total points:	30

A score of 23 in a well-educated person or a person aged less than 60 years is suggestive of cognitive impairment.

Orientation

The MMSE tests of orientation suffice most of the time, but they can be misleading where orientation to, say, date is not important to the patient. It can be helpful to ask about orientation to aspects of the environment that are more important to the patient, for example the names of nursing staff or how to get to the dining room.

Speech

Specific problems with speech can make patients seem more impaired or 'confused' than they really are. Speech disorder can mimic schizophreniform thought disorder.

Problems with speech can be divided into dysphonias (disorders of voice production, often leading to hoarse or whispered speech and abnormal cough), dysarthrias (neurological or muscular disorders of coordination of speech, leading to slurred or indistinct speech) and dysphasias (cerebral disorders leading to problems in understanding or finding words).

Dysphonias and dysarthrias can usually be distinguished from each other, and from dysphasias, on the basis of observation during the interview. The repetition of difficult word combinations ('red lorry, yellow lorry', 'baby hippopotamus') is especially problematic to people with dysarthria.

There are several dysphasic syndromes, which can broadly be divided into *fluent* and *non-fluent dysphasia*. The differences between the two are evident in spontaneous speech, and are set out in Box 4.9. The speech of people with fluent dysphasia flows normally but makes little sense. It is due to damage to Wernicke's area in the left posterior temporal region of the brain.

Speech can be further assessed by testing repetition (the ability to repeat words and phrases, for example 'cat', 'chair', 'the sun is shining', 'no ifs, ands or buts'), comprehension ('point to the door', 'take this piece of paper, fold it in half and place it on the chair next to you') and naming (point to a wristwatch and ask 'What is this called?' Then ask to name strap, face, winder, etc.). According to neurologists, it is possible to use the findings to localise problems. However, in psychiatric practice, the findings are often far from clear-cut.

Nominal dysphasia (or anomia) is of limited value in localising problems, but is useful in screening for dominant hemisphere lesions. If a speech problem is detected, a brief assessment of reading and writing should be carried out.

BOX 4.9 Fluent and Non-Fluent Dysphasia	
Fluent	**Non-fluent**
Normal rate	Slowed
Fluent	Faltering, with frustration
Syntax normal	Irregular and robotic
Prominent circumloculation and paraphasia	Problems finding nouns and verbs
	Perseveration
No insight	Insight

Attention and Concentration

The standard test of concentration is serial sevens, asking the patient to start with one hundred, subtract seven and state the answer, take seven from that and so on. The accuracy and speed of response are both relevant. The problem with this test is that it is daunting for many people, and patients often refuse even to attempt it. On the other hand, when the patient carries out the task very rapidly, it can test the doctor's own powers of concentration to destruction. Serial threes, from 20, can be used as an alternative, but, generally speaking, asking the patient to recite the months of the year backwards or to spell WORLD backwards is better tolerated and more illuminating. Letter fluency ('How many words can you think of beginning with the letter C?') and digit span (ask the patient to remember a five-figure number, then six, then seven … but not your own mobile phone number) are also useful. All of these tests can be affected by problems with specific functions such as dysphasia.

Memory

Everyone knows that memory impairment is a feature of dementia. Consequently, evidence of memory impairment causes considerable concern amongst patients and their families. However, memory impairment is commonly a consequence of difficulties with concentration, and apparently impaired memory requires careful evaluation. Patients should be warned that you are about to test memory, and encouraged to make an effort with the task. The understanding of memory is still developing and changing. Box 4.10 sets out a basic classification of memory. Those items marked with an asterisk are worth testing routinely.

Short- and long-term verbal memory are tested in the three objects test in the MMSE (Box 4.8, items 3 and 5). Remote episodic memory becomes apparent during history taking. Recent episodic memory can be tested by asking questions such as 'What is my name/job?' (provided you have introduced yourself properly), 'What has been in the news lately?' or 'What did you have for breakfast?' Of course, for the last type of question to be useful, you have to have access to a reliable informant account. Questions about the news need to be relevant to the patient's interests, and it can be helpful to remain in touch with sport results and the plot lines of TV soaps.

Confabulation occurs where the patient fills in the gaps in their episodic memory by making things up in order to maintain a continuous personal narrative. This appears to be for their own benefit, in other words, it seems to be unconscious rather than intentional.

BOX 4.10 Memory

Explicit memory (memories within conscious awareness)

- Short-term (lasts only a few seconds)
  - * Verbal (short-term memory for spoken information)
  - * Spatial (short-term memory for spatial information)
- Long-term (all other explicit memory)
  - * Episodic (personally experienced events)
  - * Semantic (facts)

Implicit memory (memories outside of conscious awareness)

- Conditioning (conditioned reflexes)
- Priming (unconscious cues to memory)
- Motor skills (e.g. driving a car)

Confabulation is said to be associated with Korsakoff's syndrome (profound short-term memory (STM) impairment without other cognitive impairments, usually a long-term consequence of either thiamine deficiency or carbon monoxide poisoning), but it can occur in all forms of STM impairment. The false account of events is often highly plausible, and the STM problem may only be evident on formal memory testing or because of conflicting accounts of events. It is entirely distinct from *pseudologica fantastica*, the telling of highly complex lies, which is a deliberate behaviour, nearly always associated with severe personality disorder. It is seen, for example, in Munchausen syndrome.

Semantic memory is traditionally tested by a set of questions such as 'What were the dates of the First World War?' 'Who is the prime minister?' and 'What is the capital of France?' Questions must be adjusted for educational level and subculture. The above questions may be part of the fundamental knowledge base for a middle-class professional, but they are likely to be completely outside of the awareness of a poorly educated disaffected teenager, currently resident in a young offenders' institution.

Abstract Thinking

Abstract thinking is frequently impaired in dementia and where there is frontal lobe damage. However, it is one of the highest-level cerebral functions, and many other factors can impair it, including psychosis and anxiety. It is usually only worth testing abstract thinking where an organic problem is suspected and the patient is reasonably relaxed.

The two traditional tests are proverb interpretation and similarities/differences. Proverb interpretation is the less useful of the two. When asked 'What is meant by "people who live in glass houses shouldn't throw stones"?', a very large proportion of the general population reply, 'Well, they'll break the windows'. It can be surprisingly difficult to judge the degree of abstraction involved in a specific answer. Some otherwise unimpaired people make interpretations of proverbs that seem to be complete *non sequiturs*, as the abstraction has lost contact with the content. In any case, interpretation of proverbs is culture bound, and potentially misleading when applied to people from ethnic minorities. The proverb most commonly used in this test is 'Too many cooks spoil the broth'.

Similarities/differences is altogether more useful. The patient is asked 'What are the similarities between a chair and a table?' and 'What are the differences between a child and a dwarf?' Abstract thinking depends on recognition of categorical similarities and differences, rather than concrete features such as 'They both have four/two legs'.

Judgement

Judgement is a specific aspect of abstract thought. Impaired judgement is obvious and alarming to those around the patient, but it is hard to test clinically. The patient is normally unaware of it. The degree of impaired judgement that leads to extravagant gambling losses may not be evident to a psychiatrist who does not know the patient. Consequently, it is most easily assessed through the history given by family and friends. The usual clinical test is to give the patient a scenario involving a judgement and asking them what they would do if, for example, 'You are in a crowded pub and you notice that a flat screen television has caught fire'. The assessment of the patient's response is subjective, and it is best to be cautious about the reliability of this kind of test, unless the response is grossly abnormal.

Parietal Lobe Tests

The dominant and non-dominant parietal lobes have different functions. Dominant parietal lobe functions can be tested more reliably than non-dominant. The overlapping pentagons test in the MMSE (Box 4.8, item 11) tests for constructional dyspraxia, which is a dominant parietal lobe sign. The patient can also be asked to draw a house. An oversimplified drawing indicates a dominant lesion; an exploded drawing may be due to a non-dominant lesion. Box 4.11 sets out some more specific parietal lobe tests.

BOX 4.11 Parietal Lobe Tests

Dominant parietal lobe tests

- Finger agnosia: Ask the patient to name which finger you touched. Touch two fingers on each side.
- Left–right disorientation: Ask the patient to put their right hand on the desk, then remove it. Repeat with left hand, then right hand again.
- Praxis: Ask the patient to mime how they would comb their hair, use scissors, clean their teeth, blow out a match. Watch for inability to do these and also for use of body parts as objects (e.g. cleans teeth with a finger).
- Calculation: Ask patient to write down five numbers and add them up.
- Writing: Ask patient to write a sentence.

Non-dominant parietal lobe tests

- Postural arm drift: Ask patient to hold out the arms, palms down, eyes closed. Watch for drift of either hand downwards. Arm drift indicates contralateral parietal lobe abnormality.
- Unilateral neglect: Ask patient, eyes closed, to tell you which hand you touched. Touch left, right, both together.

BOX 4.12 Frontal Lobe Tests

- *Grasp reflex*: Test by stroking both the patient's palms. An abnormal response is a reflex grasp of the stroking fingers.
- *Motor sequencing*: Test by asking the patient to watch what you do and copy. Then, with arms outstretched, palms down, alternate opening and closing fists, so that, as one fist opens the other closes. Alternatively, use the Luria test: tap on the desk in a repeating sequence of closed fist on desk, edge of open hand on desk, palm down on desk. Repeat Fist, Edge, Palm several times and ask patient to copy.
- *Perseveration*: Ask patient to tap three times on the table with their middle finger.
- *Alternating frames of reference*: Ask patient to tap once on the table when you tap once. Then to tap twice when you tap twice. Then to tap twice when you tap once. Then to tap once when you tap twice.

Frontal Lobe Tests

Box 4.12 sets out some reliable tests for frontal lobe dysfunction, but they are relatively insensitive, which is to say, the dysfunction has to be severe before the test becomes abnormal.

Perseveration is a frontal lobe sign, which can manifest itself either in speech or in behaviour. It consists of inappropriate repetition. The person seems unable to shift to a new frame of reference. At one end of the spectrum it may involve the repetitive use of a word far beyond its meaning (for example, a 93-year-old man from Benfleet, Essex, who, in reply to direct questions, said he had fought in Benfleet during the Korean War and that he smoked Benfleet cigarettes), and, at the other end of the spectrum, may manifest itself as continual repetition of complex behaviours such as shopping, to the extent that the patient's house fills up with decomposing fruit and vegetables. Like many other signs, it may be more obvious from the history, or in conversation, than on formal testing.

Catastrophic Reactions

The range of cognitive tests described here is quite daunting. Some patients, struggling to cope with cognitive tests, suddenly become very distressed or angry. This ends the interview in most cases, and also affects the patient's relationship with the doctor. It is not always possible to spot a catastrophic reaction developing. Reassurance and an awareness of the patient's reaction to poor performance (or sometimes to the process of being tested in itself) is important. The risk of a catastrophic reaction dictates that cognitive testing usually is best conducted towards the end of the interview.

Main Points in This Chapter

1. All psychiatric disorders can be mimicked by physical problems.
2. An awareness of the patient's experience of the interview is just as important for people with cognitive impairment as for anybody else.
3. History taking and observation throughout the interview are more important in assessing cognitive problems than specific tests.
4. Psychiatric illness impairs performance in cognitive tests.
5. It is worth learning the Mini-Mental State Examination items and a few other reliable cognitive tests. These should be practised regularly.

In the UK, one-to-one interviewing is no longer the dominant model of interaction between psychiatrists and patients. Psychiatrists increasingly work as part of multidisciplinary teams, away from the traditional office setting. For some, supporting and supervising other professionals has become as important in their work as face-to-face contact with patients. Other psychiatrists work exclusively with people who are acutely unwell, either in their own homes or in inpatient units. Nonetheless, the core skills of a psychiatrist are based upon the ability to work one-to-one, and many important issues are most easily understood in the office setting.

This section deals with key principles and concepts through exploration of the one-to-one interview

5 Office-Based Psychiatric Assessment

It is said that in football, everything is complicated by the presence of the opposing team. A very similar principle applies in clinical interviews. The technical tasks outlined in Section 1 are quite complicated, but what really makes the situation demanding is the presence of the patient, who is likely to have unpredictable expectations and needs. There are some key tasks that have to be carried out in any successful assessment interview.

Firstly, and perhaps most importantly, the psychiatrist has to establish the foundations of a relationship with the patient. It is self-evident that a good relationship with the patient is desirable, and that symptom relief (let alone recovery) is unlikely against the backdrop of a poor relationship. What is less obvious is the exact nature of a good relationship, as it does not necessarily involve doing everything the patient wants.

Secondly, a large amount of historical information has to be collected and organised, whilst carefully observing the patient and carrying out a mental state examination.

Thirdly, the psychiatrist must arrive at both a diagnosis and a thorough understanding of the patient's problems and the context within which they have arisen. This includes an assessment of risk. In combination, these make up a formulation.

Fourthly, all of this has to be explained to the patient in a form that they can understand.

Finally, the psychiatrist has to decide what interventions are likely to be helpful, negotiate a treatment plan with the patient, and persuade them to follow it.

Fortunately, these tasks overlap with each other. For example, in forming a relationship with the patient, the psychiatrist learns something about their social interactions. The process of assessment can have a powerful, though non-specific, impact on the patient's distress. It is the psychiatrist's responsibility to maximise the chances that this impact is positive rather than negative.

Like driving a motor vehicle on the road for the first time, when you start out doing psychiatric assessments, everything seems frighteningly complex. Before very long, multiple tasks are carried out simultaneously without difficulty. Or at least, this is how it is most of the time.

In trying to understand what goes on between psychiatrists and their patients, it is helpful to think about the different agendas they bring to the interview, and how the conflicting demands of these agendas can be resolved.

Dr Coltrane and Mrs Mitchell

Let us take the example of Dr Coltrane, an experienced psychiatrist, who is asked by a GP to assess Mrs Mitchell. The referral letter states that Mrs Mitchell is anxious and depressed and that she has expressed suicidal ideas.

Mrs Mitchell

Mrs Mitchell is 40 years old, and she is very unhappy. She is irritable and she has been shouting at her family a lot. Sometimes, she bursts into tears without warning. She is constantly tired but she cannot sleep at night. She has stopped going out with her friends, and she cannot be bothered with her appearance. She often wears pyjamas all day.

Her husband is fed up with trying to find out what is wrong with her. One evening they have an argument. Mrs Mitchell ends up in tears, and, in a mood of self-recrimination, says that the family would be better off if she killed herself. Her husband is alarmed and insists that she makes an appointment with their GP.

After a sympathetic but brief chat, her GP prescribes an antidepressant. Mrs Mitchell has read about these drugs, 'happy pills' that are addictive and have lots of side effects. She hesitates to take the tablets, and throws them away after a few days. She returns to see her GP a few weeks later, where she sobs uncontrollably. She tells him about her suicidal thoughts. He suggests that it might be helpful to see a psychiatrist, and she tearfully acquiesces. Although she does not say so, she is distressed by the suggestion.

On the day of the appointment, she does not want to attend. Her husband loses his temper and angrily tells her that she is going mental and needs sorting out, before she sends him mental as well. With great reluctance, she keeps the appointment.

All interviews between doctors and patients are skewed and follow rules that are very different from other types of interactions. Ordinary social reciprocity is suspended. Doctors are permitted to behave in unusual ways and to ask intrusive questions on the understanding that the relationship has a primary orientation towards the patient's needs, physical or emotional. This one-sided nature imparts much to the therapeutic potency of the relationship, but it also has a darker aspect. There is a steep power-gradient between a doctor and a patient. Even the most articulate, well-informed patient (for example, a doctor seeing his own GP) is at a disadvantage because of this power imbalance. Patients are very aware of this, and it accounts for a lot of the defensive and awkward behaviour that doctors dislike so much.

It is hard for doctors to stay in touch with the stressful quality of medical interviews, because they spend so much of their time in them. They are part of the fabric of their daily life, and they become banal. It is easy to lose sight of the fact that, whilst the doctor knows exactly how an interview is likely to proceed, many patients do not know what to expect, have little control over the situation, and so become intensely anxious. Amongst medical interviews, a first meeting with a psychiatrist is especially stressful, because of patients' preconceptions.

Preconceptions

Most psychiatrists are well aware that they are ordinary people, with no special insights into the human condition. Indeed, a belief that you have special powers of understanding or healing is incompatible with safe psychiatric practice. The general population, on the other hand, tends to experience psychiatrists as very unusual and somewhat scary people. Mrs Mitchell has never met a psychiatrist before. Like everyone else, she is influenced by innumerable jokes, films and news stories. Even broadsheet journalists struggle to distinguish psychiatrists from psychoanalysts, psychologists and psychotherapists. Popular images of psychiatrists tend to fall into two categories, the inept bleeding-heart liberal and the sinister manipulative malefactor. Both stereotypes carry an implication that psychiatrists are personally suffering from a covert madness. These are powerful images that create frightening expectations.

The popular stereotypes are probably not just the consequence of a persistently bad press. Compared with other people, psychiatrists do have a real ability to penetrate the mind, to seek out people's most private fears and to detect weaknesses. They have mastery over 'insanity', an archaic term for a mythical state that still causes fear in twenty-first century urban society as one of the worst things that can happen to you.

On first meeting a psychiatrist, either socially or professionally, many people will express their fears quite directly. This usually takes the form of a nervous joke on the theme 'I suppose you can read my inner thoughts'. Realistically, psychiatrists do have considerable legal powers to interfere in their patient's life. Most patients, attending for the first time, have no way of judging whether a psychiatrist will regard them as in need of compulsory admission to hospital. Community-based psychiatry is still relatively new. It only emerged on a significant scale in the 1980s. For many ordinary people, the memory of the forbidding asylum is very much alive, and with it the fear of indefinite incarceration. It is easy to understand why many patients approach psychiatrists for the first time with great anxiety. Often only desperation or duress drives them to attend their appointment.

The psychiatric mystique does have a few redeeming features. It gives the initial interview an impact beyond a routine medical appointment. The interview is likely to have a watershed quality. This can reinforce helpful aspects of the interaction, though equally, if you are insensitive to the patient's fears, the experience can be anxiety provoking and unhelpful.

Sitting in the waiting room, Mrs Mitchell would not be able to explain why she feels so anxious. She is unclear as to what will take place in the interview, and she has no great certainty that it will be helpful.

Agendas

Psychiatrists and patients commence interviews with separate agendas, each of which includes items that are explicit and other items that are implicit. A patient's list of questions about medication is an example of an explicit agenda item. If the patient leaves the room without having tackled those matters that were important to her at the beginning of the interview, it is certain she will feel dissatisfied. She will probably feel that she has not been understood and that this doctor is unlikely to help her. She may well not come back for follow-up appointments. On the other hand, a doctor's need for the patient to like him or her is an example of an implicit (and perhaps unconscious) agenda item.

Ultimately, it is the psychiatrist's responsibility to control the interview so that the patient is likely to benefit from it. Consequently, it is inevitable that the psychiatrist's agenda is dominant. However, both agendas create legitimate demands within the interview. It is certainly not possible simply to state each agenda at the outset in a straightforward way. Resolving the tension caused by the differences between the separate agendas is not necessarily difficult, but it does require an awareness that such agendas exist.

Mrs Mitchell's Agenda

Clearly, any individual patient's agenda is idiosyncratic, but there are themes that are common. In Mrs Mitchell's case:

1. She is worried that she might be going mad. Her current feelings and behaviour are out of character, and she cannot understand what is happening to her. Her husband and her GP both seem to think that she has a mental problem.

2. There are some behaviours that are particularly worrying her. She is very bothered by her inability to sleep. Her constant shouting at the children makes her feel bad about herself. Sometimes she worries that she could completely lose control and assault them. She has thoughts that everyone would be better off if she killed herself, and the prospect of simply not feeling anything is attractive. She knows that her suicide would be very painful for her family, but she worries that the urge might overwhelm her.

3. There are some matters that she actively wishes to conceal from the psychiatrist. The family receives state benefit payments, but both she and her husband do casual work to supplement this income. Although the sums of money are small, this is illegal and there is a well-publicised and aggressive agency that investigates benefit fraud. The family needs the extra money, but she feels guilty about breaking the law, and she is fearful of the shame of being discovered. On top of this, she has guilty feelings and regrets over a termination of pregnancy in her teens. Both of these guilty secrets are relevant to her current distress.

4. She wants the psychiatrist to explain what is wrong with her. This is not the same as being given a diagnosis. When her GP told her that she was depressed, this conveyed little information to her. She has felt 'depressed' before, but her present condition is quite different. It is a lot worse. The distinction between feeling down and having a depressive illness is not an idea that is familiar to her. She needs an explanation in terms that she can understand and accept.

5. In addition to an explanation, she wants a plan of help that makes sense to her. Just as the explanation of what is wrong must be plausible in her own terms, the treatment plan must seem credible to her.

6. Above all, she wishes to avoid adverse consequences, such as hospitalisation or the removal of her children from her care.

Dr Coltrane's Agenda

The psychiatrist's agenda is not necessarily any more straightforward than the patient's:

1. He has an initial hypothesis about Mrs Mitchell's problem, based upon the GP's letter. He wants to test and elaborate this hypothesis.

2. He wants to complete the five tasks set out at the beginning of this chapter. Ideally, he wants it all completed in the first interview, so that there are no awkward loose ends to sort out later.

3. He wants to achieve this within a specific time frame, because running late has consequences for other people, makes him feel stressed, and can lead to him missing his lunch. As patients sometimes want to talk about matters that he thinks are off the point, he wants to control the interview.

4. He is curious about the patient and he wants her to leave the interview feeling that he has helped her. If Dr Coltrane did not have such motivations, he would not want to work as a psychiatrist.

5. He wants to make sure that it is very unlikely that the patient will go on to do something untoward, such as harming herself or someone else. Such an event would affect his

professional self-esteem, but it would also have more tangible consequences, as it is likely he would be called to account for his assessment and decisions.

6. He wants to protect himself emotionally. He works with distressed people every day, and he must remain empathetic without becoming distressed himself. Distress is infectious and sometimes patients' problems resonate with problems in Dr Coltrane's life. He wants to preserve a proper professional distance between the patient and himself. He wants to avoid making disclosures about himself or being drawn into an overly friendly relationship. These issues of boundary setting are dealt with in Chapter 6.

A Basic Interview Framework

Being a skilled interviewer involves a lot more than the use of a set of behavioural procedures. There are many different ways of conducting a good interview. Everyone has their own style, determined by their personality and modified by expertise and experience. There is no script for a perfect interview. However, the behavioural procedures, which are simple and quite well known, are very useful.

Interviews move between distinct phases. An awareness of these basics facilitates the interview, and the reconciliation of agendas.

Before the Interview

Even before the interview starts, the doctor will have formed an impression of the likely nature of the problem, based on the referral letter. Over time, psychiatrists become increasingly skilled at spotting patterns and gleaning information from such letters, despite the fact that they are often brief. You learn about the fine-grained demography of the area that you work in, and the likely lifestyle of people living in particular streets. There are types of patients who are drawn to individual GPs, and there are types of referral that each GP tends to make. Taken alongside age, gender and the main symptoms, a preliminary guess about the nature of the problem is more likely to be right than wrong. Such assumptions are likely to be present, whether or not one makes them explicit.

This creates a trap before the interview has even started. Unless these assumptions are formed into an explicit hypothesis that can be tested and pursued, initial assumptions can undermine the objectivity of the assessment. They can drive a process whereby you find what you are looking for and fail to spot that which you do not expect. Hypothesising starts before the interview. Psychiatrists explicitly state to themselves what they expect to find.

There is a second pre-interview discipline that is helpful in a wide variety of circumstances. This is to be clear why you are seeing the patient and what this particular interview is for. The question may seem inane, but patients are referred for a variety of reasons. Clarity over the purpose of the interview is especially important when working in teams and in follow-up appointments, but it has usefulness in assessments too. For example, are you providing an opinion or deciding whether to take the patient on for treatment? Do the patient and the referrer have the same expectation of the assessment process? If you assume that, for example, all assessment interviews necessarily lead to follow-up until the point of recovery, clinics will contain a significant number of compliant but puzzled patients who do not want, or need, to be seen.

Office layout is worth thinking about, although offices are often shared and have multiple functions. Interviewing across a desk is intimidating, and it is better to have the patient at the side of the desk. Chairs should, wherever possible, be at the same height. Armchairs create informality, but they tend to be low, and can cause problems to older people and those with physical disabilities. The doctor and patient should be able to escape from the room unimpeded and have the means to raise the alarm if necessary (these measures are very rarely needed, but when they are, they are very important). Other staff should know whether interruptions are permitted or not.

Introductions

Introductions are a courtesy that most people recognise as important in social or business settings. Unfortunately, doctors often neglect them in their work. This is a serious error. If the start of the meeting is socially gauche, the patient will not feel comfortable in talking freely about sensitive and private matters.

Dr Coltrane goes to the waiting room, introduces himself by name and invites Mrs Mitchell to his office. He could ask the receptionist to send the patient in, but a more personal approach is less intimidating. If the opportunity arises, shaking hands with the patient is a good idea. In British culture, failing to shake hands on first meeting can carry an aloof implication about relative social status. Shaking hands implies that you are taking the other person seriously. Unfortunately, there is a critical moment for handshakes, after which it becomes unhelpfully awkward, and the moment is easily missed.

Once alone in the office, a few moments devoted to social ritual give the patient the opportunity to adjust to the setting and to the doctor as a person. Dr Coltrane indicates which chair Mrs Mitchell should sit on. He closes the door. The doctor may know that the interview will not be overheard if the door is left ajar, but the patient cannot be certain of this. He explains that he is a consultant psychiatrist and that he is seeing her at her GP's request. In other words, he makes clear his profession, his status and why he is seeing her. Regrettably, in the twenty-first century, patients still arrive in psychiatrists' clinics unaware of these basic facts, and it is as well to be unambiguous before the interview starts. The patient who thinks he or she has been referred to a chest physician for breathlessness, rather than to a psychiatrist for panic attacks, and who realises this half way through the interview, is likely to be difficult to help.

Dr Coltrane explains that the interview will last about one hour. This is a long time for a medical interview, and patients often expect something much shorter. If Mrs Mitchell has later commitments, for example if she has to pick up the children from school, the interview will start to go wrong once she realises that time is running short. A few patients think that the interview has no time limits. In either case, it is better that there is clarity about the timescale at the outset.

Helping the Patient to Describe Their Problem

Generally speaking, a good starting point is to tell the patient what you already know from the referrer. This gives the patient a point of reference as to what you need to be told, and, if they think the referrer has misunderstood, it provides an early opportunity to say so. This is usually an exercise in précis. Simply reading out the letter, with its jargon, is generally to be avoided. 'Your GP thinks you might be psychotic' is not a good start to an interview, but 'Your GP is worried about the trouble with your neighbours' is less alarming and conveys a similar meaning. There are very few good reasons not to be frank with patients, but translation from medical to English eases communication considerably.

Dr Coltrane explains what he knows, and says 'Tell me about the problem'. He allows the patient to talk. He chooses not to make notes during the first part of the interview, remaining fully attentive until the general nature of the problem has become clear. Clinical note taking can be intrusive and some patients are perturbed by it. However, the practice of writing notes after the interview has finished invites lapses of memory. At some point in the interview, one must start making notes. It can be helpful to explain, for example, 'I'm going to write down what you've told me, so that I don't forget.' If the patient is sensitive about confidentiality and record keeping, this creates an opportunity for them to raise their concerns, and in any case makes it clear why the notes are kept and that the information is being taken seriously.

The psychiatrist's comments in the early, unstructured, part of the interview need to be fairly neutral and aimed at helping the patient to express herself. For example, Mrs Mitchell weeps and hesitates as she describes her irritability, how she shouts at the children and how they become upset. There are a number of clichéd stock phrases used by generations of psychiatrists, which continue to work in helping patients to talk about difficult matters, for example:

> *'It's ok to cry'*
> *'That sounds very difficult'*
> *'That seems to be worrying you'*
> *'Take your time telling me about it'*

Similarly, if the patient cries, the offer of a box of tissues acknowledges the patient's distress, without implying that the doctor cannot cope with it. It is a mistake to try and stop the patient from crying or being upset, as this will lead the interview away from important material.

If the patient is not expressing herself clearly, it is possible to clarify without becoming prematurely directive:

Dr Coltrane: *'Can I just check I've understood this correctly? Things were OK until about nine months ago, around the time your friend was diagnosed with cancer. Things got worse in March when you had a sudden feeling that you were about to die when you were out shopping. After that, you became generally more tense and anxious, and you started sleeping badly. More recently you've become tearful and very low in mood.'*

This is a capsule summary, organising and feeding back part of the story. If the doctor has it right, the interview can move on and the patient knows she has been heard. If it is wrong, the patient can correct the summary. In either case, the patient knows that the doctor is taking the trouble to understand properly. The length of the initial, unstructured, part of the interview depends upon whether one feels that cogent information is emerging. Occasionally, a patient will give a full and well-organised history spontaneously. This is rare. Most people, when talking about themselves, will eventually wander and start to interdigitate themes. This is hard for the listener to follow (we have all had this experience when cornered at parties). At this point, the doctor must intervene.

Hypothesis Testing

By now, the psychiatrist will either have a more complicated version of his initial hypothesis or a completely new hypothesis about the nature of the problem. The next, more directive, phase of the interview aims both to test the hypothesis and to fill out the overall picture. This means asking about symptoms that have not been volunteered: both symptoms that are normally expected, in keeping with the hypothesis (in Mrs Mitchell's case loss of appetite, diurnal variation of mood, impaired concentration, etc.) and symptoms associated with alternative explanations (in Mrs Mitchell's case, long-standing phobic symptoms and obsessional symptoms). Throughout, Dr Coltrane attempts to relate symptoms to antecedents, for example by asking about stresses in Mrs Mitchell's life at the time of the onset of symptoms. He asks about alterations in behaviour consequent upon the symptoms.

Mrs Mitchell is tearful and distressed. She feels that the problem started when a close friend was diagnosed with cancer nine months earlier, but that things became much more difficult following an initial panic attack three months later. She has had these episodes regularly since, and has become increasingly distressed, irritable and sleepless. She is fearful that she is going mad.

Dr Coltrane has established through direct questions that Mrs Mitchell was already experiencing depressive symptoms prior to the onset of panic attacks, and that these are typical hyperventilatory episodes. They have continued at a rate of about three a week, with no particular precipitants, and in no particular situation. There is no true phobic avoidance, but she has generally withdrawn from her normal activities and lacks motivation. There has been a steady worsening of depressive symptoms, including tearfulness, hopelessness, sleep disturbance (waking through the night and early waking), irritability, impaired concentration with secondary forgetfulness, loss of energy, loss of motivation and loss of libido. She has a reduced appetite, and she has lost about 5 kg (11 lb) in weight. She frequently thinks of death and is concerned that she might take her own life, but she does not want to die. Her forgetfulness has led her to worry that she might have Alzheimer's disease like her grandmother.

In this case, the general nature of the problem matches Dr Coltrane's initial hypothesis, but the context and antecedents have yet to be fully explored.

Controlling the Interview

Although interviews become increasingly structured as they proceed, the need to control the interview can arise at any stage. At the simplest, digressions and repetitions must be controlled. Clarifications are necessary, and, later on, some topics can only be dealt with through direct and closed questions. As the psychiatrist fills out the history, he has to move the discussion smoothly through a range of topics, which may not appear to the patient to be logically connected.

It is easy to get the degree of control wrong. Pushing the interview on too quickly can appear dismissive, and risks overlooking important information. Lack of control, for fear of causing offence, leads to an unfocused interview, which also risks omissions.

Curtailing discussion is best done explicitly, and the degree of bluntness needed depends on the patient's responsiveness to social cues:

> 'OK, I'd like to move on to ask you about . . .'
> 'This is obviously important to you, but there are some other things I need to understand'
> 'We seem to have drifted off the point. Let's go back to what you said about . . .'
> 'Hang on, STOP, I've lost track here. Tell me about . . .'

These remarks vary in subtlety, but all are polite and signal a clear intent. Only very occasionally does the doctor have to give up and let the interview go where it will, usually with the need to bring the patient back for a second interview in order to gain more coherent information.

It is considerably easier to stop patients from talking than it is to get them to talk when they are reluctant to do so. Where a patient is hesitant, or obviously distressed, on being asked about a particular area of their life, it is usually helpful to acknowledge this. A comment such as 'You look really uncomfortable' followed by silence can allow the patient to approach the difficulty more gradually.

The process of drawing out emotionally charged information from someone has more to do with not allowing the subject to change than it has to do with questioning per se. If it becomes apparent that the patient really does not want to discuss something, you can attempt to defuse the situation and gain some information by a (somewhat disingenuous) ploy such as 'Look, you are obviously very uncomfortable with this, so don't tell me about it. Just tell me why this is difficult for you.'

A major strategy that we all use to avoid emotionally laden subjects is vagueness. Vague answers to important questions demand the use of tightly closed questions and an emphasis on specifics:

> 'When does *x* happen?'
> 'Tell me about the last time that happened'
> 'What did you do next?'
> 'OK, how much did you drink yesterday?'

Non-Verbal Communication

Within an interview, non-verbal communication is important, both in assessing the patient and as a tool for the doctor. Patients communicate their state of ease or distress in the here and now mainly non-verbally, for example by facial expression, by maintaining or avoiding eye contact, by adopting different postures and so on. Because all communication is reciprocal, the doctor automatically responds non-verbally (or appears robotic if he does not).

Attention to the patient's non-verbal behaviour is part of mental state examination, but it also reflects how the patient experiences the interview. The tense, uneasy patient needs more social introduction at the start of the interview than someone who is obviously more composed. Non-verbal clues signal the affect associated with different subjects and may mark areas where the patient has significant problems, but has difficulty in saying so.

There are some non-verbal tools at the interviewer's disposal that can be used to control the interview. They are, principally, gestures aimed at encouraging the patient to talk, gestures aimed at holding close attention on a particular subject, and those aimed at closing off a particular subject. The gestures are familiar from ordinary social intercourse. One's skill in using them professionally depends largely on possession of the corresponding social skills in ordinary life (although, like many other things, social skills can sometimes be faked).

Encouraging the patient to talk freely rests on an impression of interest and an illusion of unhurriedness. Gestures therefore indicate that the doctor is relaxed, for example moving back from the desk and adopting an 'open' body posture. Discarding the case notes temporarily and with some deliberation, though quasi-theatrical, can give a message of particular attention. This type of manoeuvre allows the maintenance of eye contact.

Holding the focus on a particular topic involves further gestures of attention. Abandonment of the case notes and close eye contact apply here too, though open body postures are less useful. On the contrary, leaning forward and refusing to relax a body posture discourages a shift away from the subject. This may involve overriding the patient's body language of discomfort. It is a fine judgement how far to sustain this. If overdone, it can create the appearance of a maniacally staring-eyed, hunched psychiatrist, which may confirm the patient's worst fears.

'Closing off' gestures may be the converse of the above, or may involve a more positive and deliberate action. Picking up the case notes again indicates an alteration in the interview, as does reversion to a closed posture. Winding up or summarising comments are usefully accompanied by corresponding hand movements. An open palmed gesture is a clear signal to stop.

The Structured Part of the Interview

Very few people have a clear understanding of the way in which contextual factors provoke and shape their mental illness. Drawing out this narrative is a powerful, but non-specific, therapeutic factor in psychiatric interviewing. By moving systematically through the standard structure of the psychiatric history (set out in Chapter 3), contextual factors become apparent. If the relationship between patient and psychiatrist is developing satisfactorily, then issues that the patient never intended to mention, such as Mrs Mitchell's worries over benefit fraud, may be disclosed. Essentially, the patient decides that the psychiatrist is trustworthy. Even where difficult material is not immediately volunteered, there are often clues in the history or in the patient's response to particular types of questions. Attentiveness to clues, gaps and bits of history that do not make sense is what allows psychiatrists to uncover the most difficult parts of patients' stories.

Recording the history as a time line, a strict chronology, will reveal relationships between events. Gaps in the chronology should be explored, as they can mark important secrets, such as periods of imprisonment. Current preoccupations can offer clues to important past events. Mrs Mitchell's guilt over benefits, and fear of loss with respect to her friend, both have a thematic link with her unresolved feelings over the termination of pregnancy. Questions about other things that make her feel guilty or other difficult losses in her life may well lead to a disclosure.

There is a caveat here. Forced disclosure is not a legitimate part of an assessment interview, and it requires a fine judgement to decide how hard to push patients on issues that distress them. It can be tempting to guess what lies behind a patient's distress, and to put the guess to them. This is not a good idea, as patients sometimes agree to suggested histories that are not correct and, in extreme cases, may be persuaded of their veracity.

By working his way through the history, and completing those relevant parts of mental state examination omitted earlier, Dr Coltrane comes to an initial assessment of Mrs Mitchell's problem. This is still a hypothesis, because the process of hypothesising is never truly completed. New information can always emerge. You become incrementally more certain, but never unshakably so.

Mrs Mitchell is a woman with an anxious, perfectionist personality. She is religious, and has high moral expectations of herself. She had a termination of pregnancy in her teens, which is the subject of continuing guilt. Her best friend had a hysterectomy for cervical carcinoma nine months ago, and Mrs Mitchell worries that she will die. She has become increasingly concerned about her own health. The couple have debts, which is why they take casual work. Forgetfulness and the onset of panic attacks exacerbated her fears over physical health, and rising anxiety provoked further panic. Her anxiety, depression and irritability have led to a deterioration in her marriage, making her feel worse about herself, and hence more depressed. She worries that she may hit the children and that they may be taken out of her care. She also worries that she will take her own life, and that the children's lives will be blighted.

No single factor has directly caused her current misery, but when taken together in the context of her life, it is understandable how these stresses have come together at this time with a consequent reaction of a moderately severe depression with secondary anxiety.

Reassurance

Some of Mrs Mitchell's initial agenda items invite a response of reassurance. Her fear that she has dementia was raised early on. Towards the end of the interview, Dr Coltrane had sufficient history to decide that her forgetfulness was due to impaired concentration. He could truthfully reassure her.

Not all such fears are so easily dealt with. Mrs Mitchell's fear of hospitalisation was also expressed early in the interview. Dr Coltrane already knew that it was unlikely that he would want to admit her, but it was too soon to be sure. Similarly, later on, her fear of the involvement of child protection agencies could not be immediately dealt with. It is very tempting to offer reassurance on these kinds of issues, but it is essential to be truthful. A qualified reassurance will heighten rather than relieve anxieties ('Your children will probably not get taken away'). The habit of premature reassurance inevitably leads eventually to betrayal. Someone will prove to pose a higher risk than one initially supposed. All that the psychiatrist can do is to acknowledge the patient's anxiety, and promise to return to the subject at the end of the interview. There is a real dilemma over how much reassurance to give, and if in doubt, it is best to explicitly delay the question until the end of the assessment.

Closing the Interview

Interviews need proper endings. Hopefully, the movement between free discussion and direct questioning, giving feedback through capsule summaries, the systematic exploration of context and attentiveness to clues has allowed Dr Coltrane to deal with his own agenda whilst allowing Mrs Mitchell to disclose hers. At the end of the interview, Dr Coltrane checks that Mrs Mitchell does not hold undisclosed information or agenda items. The closing question, 'Is there anything else that you feel it is important for me to know?' regularly reveals significant information and concerns. This can provoke a complete re-evaluation of the assessment. (It is similarly helpful at the end of follow-up appointments to ask 'Is there anything else you wanted to discuss?' Quite apart from ensuring thoroughness, such questions give an impression of unhurriedness.)

Dr Coltrane feeds back his assessment to Mrs Mitchell, a full (rather than a capsule) summary. He is more or less obliged to give the patient a diagnosis, or at least a reframing of the problem as seen through his eyes. At this stage, the diagnosis or formulation is not always comprehensive or definitive. However, the patient wants to know what the doctor makes of her. It is a major agenda item. Such an explanation has to be both comprehensible and plausible to the patient. There is little point in telling someone with no psychiatric knowledge that they have a depressive illness without further explanation. It is more useful to explain that these particular symptoms are common, that they generally come as a group and that they are all part of depression. This is an illness insofar as it continues under its own momentum, even after the stresses that initially caused it have stopped. This is both in keeping with the psychiatric concept of the illness, and it is likely to make sense to Mrs Mitchell.

Main Points in This Chapter

1. Clinical interviewing is one of the main tools of the psychiatrist. Assessment interviews are daunting and strange to patients. They are more than an exercise in information gathering.
2. Patients and doctors enter clinical interviews with separate agendas. Each of them has preconceptions, which substantially affect the nature of the interview.
3. Both agendas are valid, but there is a tension between them. The main points in each agenda must be dealt with in the course of the interview.
4. Interviews move between different stages, which require different techniques.
5. Interviews are essentially interactive. Understanding the patient's experience of the interview assists the doctor in his or her task.
6. Assessment develops through hypothesis formation and testing.

Understanding and Managing Relationships with Patients

Interactions between psychiatrists and their patients occur in the context of a therapeutic relationship. Sometimes the relationship is very brief. Sometimes the relationship lasts for many years. These relationships can go wrong. When they do, the problem usually has its origin in the beginning of the relationship, but only becomes evident far later.

All doctors have a responsibility to contain their relationship with their patient within distinct boundaries. This is a legal and ethical obligation. It is also crucial to the therapeutic effectiveness of the relationship. There are dilemmas in maintaining boundaries that cannot be resolved, but they must be actively managed. On the one hand, the doctor must be concerned for, and interested in, the patient. Doctors must be sufficiently giving of themselves so that the patient feels able to trust them. On the other hand, the doctor must maintain a professional distance and bring a dispassionate objectivity to the relationship. He or she cannot let the patient enter the doctor's personal life. He must refrain from giving advice outside of his expertise. Doctors must not let the patient's dependency grow to unmanageable proportions. Above all, they must not allow the therapeutic relationship to develop in such a way that it primarily serves their needs and not the patient's.

There are processes that operate within all therapeutic relationships that generate threats to the maintenance of appropriate boundaries. These include:

1. Transference reactions
2. Dependency
3. Identification
4. Breaches of confidentiality
5. The urge to rescue patients
6. Compromised truthfulness
7. Abuses of power

Each of these is considered below. There are also some dilemmas that commonly arise in clinical situations. These concern:

8. Gifts
9. Humour
10. Self-disclosure
11. Physical contact
12. Contact outside of the clinical setting
13. Termination

These are dealt with later in the chapter.

Transference Reactions

Transference is a concept that was developed by Sigmund Freud. It has a particular meaning and importance in psychoanalysis. However, it is a common and observable phenomenon, which is important beyond the confines of specialist psychotherapy.

The patient usually has little information about the psychiatrist. The psychiatrist knows a lot about the patient, but the reverse is not true. The patient has no knowledge of the psychiatrist's personality or their life outside of the professional role. The psychiatrist is likely to play a significant role in the patient's life, at least in the short term. It is understandable, or inevitable, that the patient is driven to try and understand the psychiatrist as a person. The gaps tend to be filled by drawing on models set by significant people in the patient's past. For example, patients sometimes respond to the psychiatrist as if he or she is a judgemental and punitive parent, and react to quite neutral remarks with a defensive truculence. This draws on an example of middle-aged authority set by their parents. The doctor may have none of these parental characteristics, but in the absence of evidence, the patient behaves as if they have. This is transference as described by Freud. In practice, it includes other elements, for example idealisation. All sorts of qualities can be attributed to the doctor in the absence of unambiguous evidence.

Dr Coltrane had a bad experience when he was 27 years old, three years through his psychiatric training. He was self-confident, and by now happy to work independently. He saw Mrs Chandler as a new outpatient. She was an attractive 34-year-old woman, with children aged 15 and 12. She had married young, and though her husband was a decent man, she had grown bored with him. When the children were small, he developed a domestic routine around the television and football, and he was content to carry on with this lifestyle now that the children were more independent. Mrs Chandler, on the other hand, was keen to have the active social life she missed when her children were young. She found a secretarial job, and flirting with the boss developed into an affair. She felt guilty about this, and she started to drink heavily. She became depressed, and eventually took a serious overdose whilst drunk.

Dr Coltrane saw her regularly in the clinic over the next few months. He helped her to stop drinking, and after some joint sessions with the couple, the marriage seemed to be improving. Mrs Chandler started to take more care over her appearance, which Dr Coltrane took to be a sign that she was less depressed. However, after an appointment when he told her that he felt she could be discharged, she confessed that she had resumed drinking. At the next appointment, she attended with her husband, who was surprised to hear about the drinking, as he had seen no evidence of it. A few weeks later, the drinking had reportedly stopped, but Mrs Chandler took a small and entirely unexpected overdose.

Eventually, Dr Coltrane told her that he was leaving his post for a similar one at a nearby hospital. Mrs Chandler told him she did not want to see another psychiatrist, and they agreed that she should be discharged. She unexpectedly turned up at his final clinic and seemed flustered. She hastily handed him a letter and left. Dr Coltrane opened the letter at lunchtime. He was shocked by its contents:

Dear Dr Coltrane
   Thank you for being a good doctor to me and helping me out of my problems in the first few months that I was seeing you. I have been misleading you recently so that you would keep seeing me. The fact is I love you, and I think that you have some feelings for me. I have sat in your

room longing to hold you. Doctors can't have relationships with patients, but I'm not your patient now. Please call this number. I'll be waiting to hear from you.
   Love Tracey

Dr Coltrane took the letter to his consultant, Dr Davis, who was amused. The reception staff at the clinic had told him some weeks before that Mrs Chandler was besotted with Dr Coltrane. He had thought that Dr Coltrane was aware of this. On Dr Davis' advice, Dr Coltrane wrote her a very dry letter explaining that patients often develop strong feelings about their doctor. He pointed out that she knew very little about him, and bluntly stated that further contact between them would be inappropriate. He suggested that, if this distressed her, she should contact Dr Davis.

The incident knocked Dr Coltrane's confidence. He felt that he had made a huge mistake, and that this was bound to have an adverse effect on the patient. He also felt oddly violated, and was very uncomfortable at receiving an unwanted and taboo sexual advance.

The problem had its origins in the fact that Dr Coltrane had rendered himself oblivious to Mrs Chandler's behaviour towards him. At the beginning he felt that Mrs Chandler was attractive, and he dealt with this by ignoring it. In his efforts to respond to the patient in an entirely non-sexual and appropriate manner, he had driven her seductiveness from his awareness.

Mrs Chandler was not a sexual predator. Grateful to be feeling better, she had idealised Dr Coltrane. Although not especially good-looking, he seemed clever and kind. She imagined he had an exciting life, free of boring domesticity. Unable to read his responses to her, and in the absence of a clear message that Dr Coltrane was not sexually available to her, she escalated her signals to the point of explicitness.

The warning signs were obvious. If he had allowed himself to spot them, Dr Coltrane could have confronted her over-attachment. Given some time, it might have been possible to manage the relationship in a therapeutic way. On the other hand, if Mrs Chandler had known a little bit more about him, her fantasies might not have run so wildly out of control. This, however, would have had implications of its own for their relationship.

Dependency

Dependency is an inevitable development in a therapeutic relationship that the patient finds helpful, and it must be properly managed. It is the converse of transference, where strong feelings about the doctor are constructed largely from the patient's fantasies. Dependency occurs as the patient gets to know the psychiatrist as a person, and comes to feel that their well-being in the real world is contingent upon contact with him or her. Knowledge of the doctor as a person makes transference problems less likely, but it promotes dependency. The problem with dependency is that it undermines the patient's confidence in their ability to find their own solutions to problems. It can be burdensome, and sometimes intrusive, for the doctor.

Mrs Redding is a 30-year-old married woman. Her husband is 15 years older, and has grown-up children from a previous relationship. The couple are childless, a vasectomy reversal having failed. Mrs Redding has suffered anxiety and episodes of low mood since her teens. She is close to her mother and sees her every day. She has always looked to her mother for advice. She is a very regular attender at her GP's surgery. One day, she consults her GP about an episode of palpitations. She has difficulty in accepting that the symptom is related to anxiety. Exasperated, the GP refers her to the local consultant psychiatrist, Dr Parker.

Dr Parker sees Mrs Redding in a busy outpatient clinic. The problem seems straightforward. Although the interview is relatively brief, he is satisfied that he has made a full assessment and established an appropriate treatment plan. He is aware that Mrs Redding is likely to remain anxious indefinitely, and he anticipates seeing her on only three or four occasions.

Although the consultation is somewhat hurried, Mrs Redding is very happy with it. She feels a good deal better immediately. Dr Parker seems to have grasped the heart of her unhappiness. She is sure he can help her. At the next appointment she reports improvement. Returning after a further month, things have deteriorated. Dr Parker explores recent events, and identifies a row with her stepdaughter as the cause of the problem. Mrs Redding finds this helpful, and feels better. A pattern in the treatment is established whereby Mrs Redding never improves for long enough for discharge. She is well satisfied with the treatment, as Dr Parker seems always to be able to understand what is bothering her.

Meanwhile, Dr Parker is happy to see Mrs Redding. She never wants much time, and she is always grateful for seeing him. He recognises that most exacerbations of symptoms are related to her inability to set limits on her stepdaughter, who abuses her hospitality and causes trouble between the couple. After unsuccessfully trying to get her to work out a strategy to deal with this, he increasingly gives direct advice on how Mr and Mrs Redding can together contain the stepdaughter's behaviour. By and large, his suggestions are effective, and the patient is so pleased that she brings other problems to Dr Parker for advice. Her husband starts deferring decisions until Dr Parker's views are known. Dr Parker is aware that Mrs Redding is dependent upon him, but a particular event makes him realise that he must do something about it.

A week after an appointment, Mr Redding phones him in his office. He tells Dr Parker that the couple really need his advice. The opportunity to move house has arisen, but they feel unable to make a final decision until they know Dr Parker's views. Will it have a good or bad effect on Mrs Redding? Naturally, Dr Parker does not know, but Mr Redding is a little put out when he declines to express an opinion.

Dr Parker is now forced to reflect properly on the state of this therapeutic relationship. He realises that Mrs Redding's anxiety symptoms are probably much as they have been for ten years. His personal involvement, far from being therapeutic, has burdened the couple with a dependency on him that has invaded their family life. It has undermined their ability to resolve difficulties and make decisions for themselves. Mrs Redding is perfectly happy with this, as it has made her feel more secure. It follows the familiar pattern of her relationship with her mother.

Dr Parker could allow things to drift on like this, but he feels that it would be irresponsible. At the next appointment, he explains to Mr and Mrs Redding what he feels has gone wrong. He makes a plan to discharge Mrs Redding after three further appointments. The couple are perturbed, but after two years of treatment, Mrs Redding is eventually discharged, reasonably happy, but with little change in symptoms.

Dr Parker is an experienced and skilled psychiatrist, but he made some errors. When he first saw her, he could have foreseen that Mrs Redding had a capacity to become very dependent. This was evident from the nature of her relationship with her mother. His first and biggest mistake occurred through haste. At the first interview, he had a clear plan for the duration of contact, but he did not clearly convey this. Within the therapeutic relationship, there was no clear treatment objective. Without this, Mrs Redding had an expectation that contact would be indefinite. For her, good relationships were characterised by dependency, and she had no way of knowing that this was inappropriate to the psychiatric setting. On the contrary, this was a particularly satisfactory dependent relationship, as Dr Parker brought an expertise and authority into her life that others lacked.

Dr Parker's second mistake was that, as he hurried through his clinics, he failed to notice that the relationship was drifting and purposeless. If he had stopped to review the situation after six months, he would have seen that he needed to take remedial action. As it was, he did not recognise this until the problem was severe.

Problems of this type are common, and they cannot always be neatly resolved. Some patients with long-term mental health problems, such as unstable bipolar disorder, need to remain in follow-up indefinitely. Treatment involves mental health professionals directly in the patient's daily life. This means working within a dependency relationship. The dependency may be passed between different individuals occupying a single professional role, for example, a community mental health nurse. These changes demand consistency with regard to professional boundaries. Failures to set boundaries are more, rather than less, damaging in these situations.

Identification

Patients are not the only ones who sometimes misconstrue therapeutic relationships. It is inevitable that psychiatrists will from time to time encounter patients with backgrounds similar to their own. The doctor and the patient may be struggling with similar problems in their personal lives. It is hard to avoid feeling a special kindred spirit with these patients. It sometimes seems that understanding the patient's situation casts a revealing light on the doctor's life. The character of clinical interviews can subtly shift away from the professional towards something resembling a friendship.

There are considerable dangers under these circumstances. Firstly, hypothesising can break down. Identification leads to a loss of objectivity, and the psychiatrist starts making assumptions about the patient. The existence of parallels does not mean that everything is the same. Testing hypotheses is more important than usual, in order to avoid mistakes in assessment.

Secondly, the relationship is no longer truly patient centred, and an ambiguity can arise as to the purpose of the therapeutic relationship. This invites all the other types of boundary problems to occur. Even if this does not happen, the therapeutic nature of the relationship is compromised.

All psychiatrists will identify with some patients at some time. This need not lead to boundary breaches, provided that the psychiatrist has a degree of self-awareness. This issue is discussed at length in Section 4.

Breaches of Confidentiality

In order to treat patients, doctors must be able to obtain sensitive personal information from them. Patients give the information on the understanding that confidentiality will be maintained. This protects the patient from the possibility that disclosures will leak out into the rest of their life, with adverse consequences.

Confidentiality is more complex than this reassuringly simple model. It is an active and dynamic issue between the doctor and the patient. In the example of the interview between

Dr Coltrane and Mrs Mitchell in Chapter 5, Mrs Mitchell was able to talk about herself knowing that doctors observe confidentiality. However, she had an implicit awareness that this confidentiality was not absolute. She was concerned that her children could be removed from her care as a consequence of her discussion with Dr Coltrane. In principle, she was correct. Where a doctor believes that a patient is seriously neglecting or abusing a child, he is obliged to override confidentiality and to take appropriate action to protect the child. This is a high-order legal and ethical obligation. Similarly, Mrs Mitchell was aware that psychiatrists can initiate admission to hospital under compulsion, which is another process that overrides confidentiality.

The awareness that confidentiality has limitations is widespread. It did not prevent Mrs Mitchell from being frank, but it did affect her agenda and the way that the interview proceeded. Patients do not imagine that confidentiality is absolute, and if they want absolute confidentiality, they will seek assurances prior to disclosures. Instead, there is an understanding that confidentiality is a high-ranking principle and that it will not be broken casually.

Confidentiality is attacked by many pressures external to the therapeutic relationship. Insurance companies, benefit agencies and others, demand information that has been given in confidence. Patients permit the release of this information under duress, as otherwise they are denied their entitlements. Confidential information is shared between doctors and other health professionals, and is recorded in systems that are not 100 per cent secure.

This emphasises the importance that individual doctors must attach to the maintenance of confidentiality at a personal level. Some psychiatric case histories make spectacular anecdotes. If such stories are related in a crowded restaurant, anyone overhearing is likely to lose faith in doctors' ability to be discreet. Within clinical teams, confidentiality issues must be constantly attended to.

Dr Parker sees a middle-aged woman with a history of childhood sexual abuse and he describes this in his letter to the GP. The GP's receptionist reads the letter. When the patient next attends the surgery, the receptionist, in a quiet and kindly way, says 'Oh Eileen, you should have told us about that terrible business when you were a child.' The patient changes GP and never returns to the psychiatric clinic.

The Urge to Rescue Patients

Many people develop mental health problems in dreadful social or emotional circumstances. Mental illness not only causes them distress, it also restricts their ability to resolve more tangible problems. Psychiatrists aim to relieve symptoms through psychological, social or pharmacological interventions. As the patient's mental state improves, they become able to act autonomously to resolve the problems in their life, which in turn reduces the stresses that exacerbate mental illness.

There is sometimes a temptation in the psychiatrist to move beyond their appropriate role, and to take on personal responsibility for rescuing the patient from their circumstances. This can take many forms. Interviewing a patient's parents and criticising them in the role of the patient's champion is not generally helpful; facilitating change within a family from a neutral position, by providing information or clarifying communication, is much more effective. There is an essential difference between ensuring that a patient claims his or her full welfare benefit entitlement and providing false information to a welfare agency, in order to help the patient to secure benefits beyond entitlement.

When you start to feel the urge to rescue the patient, there is a prima facie case that the therapeutic relationship is going wrong. Boundaries will be breached unless the psychiatrist stops to consider what it is that is driving the urge.

Compromised Truthfulness

The doctor's duty to be truthful guards a boundary, both with individual patients and with society in general. At an individual level, doctors cannot help their patients if their truthfulness is in doubt, or if they protect patients from unpalatable truths. Society trusts doctors to be truthful. A medical report carries a gravity that is contingent upon its truthfulness being beyond doubt. It may occasionally seem that compromising your truthfulness will help an individual patient, but once discovered, there is considerable damage to your individual credibility, and to the credibility of the profession as a whole.

Mr Baker, suffering from anxiety, is referred to Dr Parker. He has witnessed a homicide, and he is frightened of the consequences of giving evidence. He requests a letter to the court to say that he is too unwell to give evidence. Dr Parker declines, because it is not true. Although it will be unpleasant and frightening for Mr Baker to give evidence, he is capable of doing so. Avoidance will only worsen his anxiety. If it were to become known that Dr Parker is willing to give untruthful letters of this sort, there would be a real risk of future witnesses being intimidated into seeing him to this end.

Abuses of Power

Doctors wield power over their patients. They are well educated, well paid and they are afforded a range of privileges. Patients tend to trust them. A patient will allow a doctor to perform an intimate examination on first meeting and with minimal explanation. The patient cannot necessarily distinguish between a breast examination carried out for clinical reasons and one carried out for the doctor's sexual gratification. Nonetheless, many women will unquestioningly agree to the procedure. This combination of trust and power can be abused, sometimes with catastrophic consequences.

Dr Evans was a middle-aged psychiatrist with a drink problem. He spent his evenings drinking morosely in his study. At work, he had difficulty in adjusting to new working patterns and organisational change. He isolated himself from his colleagues and stopped attending meetings. The only part of his job that he really enjoyed was a CBT clinic that he held once a week in a local private consultation office.

Dr Evans had trained in the technique many years before, and he increasingly felt that it was important to deploy more warmth and human contact than was implied during his manualised training. Poor self-esteem and lack of self-confidence were a big problem for many patients he saw, especially the women. Sometimes he would compliment them on their appearance. He would take their hand, or touch their hair.

Some patients were obviously discomforted by his personal comments or touching, and he would desist. Others appeared confused, unsure whether to be flattered or frightened. Yet others froze and gave a misleading impression of being unperturbed. Sometimes he would tell these women that, under other circumstances, he would be very pleased to have a relationship with them himself. He kissed one woman on the lips. Before long, he kissed several of them. Occasionally, the embraces involved sexual touching, and in due course he had intercourse with a patient. A pattern became established.

Eventually, there was a complaint and an investigation. Patients came forward and gave evidence about their distress over his violations. The police were involved, but no charges were brought, because of ambiguities over consent. Dr Evans lost his job and was struck from the medical register. He told his friends that he was the victim of a campaign of vilification. He may have been unwise, he said, but at the end of the day the sex was consensual and he had done nothing wrong. He felt that some of the women had benefited from their sexual relationship with him.

This fictional story makes uncomfortable reading, and the circumstances are remote from the experience of psychiatrists in training. We include it because such occurrences are the worst possible outcome of a breach of professional boundaries. It involves an ordinary doctor, a man with problems, but not someone who set out to be a sexual predator. He drifted into a gross and inexcusable abuse of power. Patients and their families can be irretrievably damaged in such circumstances.

These incidents really do happen, often to the amazement and horror of colleagues. None of the details about Dr Evans are unrealistic. This is how some abuses of power commonly develop. Trainees, too, can run into trouble with the sexualisation of therapeutic relationships. The doctors involved rarely recognise the abuse of power involved, but it is invariable.

Two factors made Dr Evans especially dangerous. His isolation from his colleagues removed him from peer support and supervision. Everyone needs this. In its absence, he could ignore his first transgression of the boundaries, namely unprofessional personal compliments and implicitly sexual touching (hand caressing and hair stroking). His capacity for *post hoc* rationalisation allowed him to become a scheming sexual predator, whilst persuading himself and his patients that he was still acting as a caring professional.

Although other types of abuses of power are less dramatic (for example, financial dealings with patients), they frequently turn on similar dynamics and are always damaging to patients. Rationalisation of the abuse is particularly dangerous, as it is frequently the last of a series of breaches of boundaries. It allows the doctor to serve his own needs at the cost of his patients

Dilemmas in the Maintenance of Boundaries

There are a number of commonly occurring dilemmas, which highlight the difficult judgements that must be made in guarding the boundaries of the therapeutic relationship.

Gifts

Patients frequently offer psychiatrists gifts as a token of gratitude for their help. In other walks of life, this is unremarkable. For the psychiatrist, accepting a gift from a patient creates a real dilemma. Patients often offer a small and inexpensive gift at the end of a successful treatment. It has an importance for them as a social ritual, marking the end of a relationship that has resolved a problem for them. It creates a balance in a situation where there was a skew. The doctor has given something to them, and they have given something back. It allows them to part as a restored social equal. Refusal of such a gift causes offence and mars the termination of treatment.

Some patients offer gifts that are extravagant or excessively personal. Others give gifts regularly. Accepting these gifts is problematic. Mostly, patients give them because they like their doctor, but there may be other motives and other meanings. Some patients seek to create an indebtedness or special status for themselves, to be cashed in at a later time. Some patients are attempting to enter the doctor's personal life. Some insecure patients feel that gifts are needed to retain a relationship with the doctor. The gift symbolises a developing problem in the relationship.

In all cases, the doctor has to consider why this patient is offering a gift at this time. He or she must be prepared to discuss this with the patient. Inappropriate gifts should be refused, even if the patient is insistent. Most employers have policies forbidding the acceptance of any but the most trivial gifts, and the patient should be told this. Most importantly, you should never imagine that accepting a gift is of no significance. The doctor must always try to understand what it means.

Humour

Laughter and humour are important parts of discourse. They can defuse tensions, they can be used to vividly illustrate a point, and they can improve rapport within a relationship. Within teams they can improve morale and team spirit, and act as a foil to the grimness of some aspects of psychiatric work.

However, humour often has a hostile edge; someone is the butt of it. Laughter at what a patient has said may be offered warmly by the doctor, but may be taken as derisive or dismissive by the patient. Anxious and depressed patients may be unable to grasp the point of a joke, leaving both doctor and patient feeling awkward. A humorous remark reveals a lot about the teller's underlying values and beliefs, and once these are exposed, they may irreversibly change the relationship with the patient. The doctor's position of non-judgemental neutrality is important to the patient's willingness to expose their most private concerns, and once this position is lost, it cannot be recovered. Most humour has an element of ambiguity or wordplay, which psychotic or paranoid patients are likely to misinterpret. In teams, humour can run out of control, and teasing can proceed to bullying. An impression of flippancy can develop. Laughter and humour are powerful tools. They must be treated with respect, as they can cause harm.

Self-Disclosure

Patients grow curious about their psychiatrist, especially if they have known them for a long time. They piece together facts learnt from other patients and from overheard conversations. It can be alarming to discover that a lot of information about you is in the public domain. This is compounded by the Internet, which places everyone on public display.

On meeting, a new patient says that you have treated his aunt for years, that she says you are very nice, that he gathers you are married with two children and that you support Manchester City Football Club. He is a United fan himself. It later emerges that he knows that you are an atheist, whereas he is a Catholic. None of this is a disaster for the therapeutic relationship, but it does mean that you are not starting with a blank sheet. There are some potential issues that may arise later, for example he may feel unable to comfortably discuss some worries he has about his social contacts at the church, feeling that you will not understand.

This process of prior knowledge cannot be prevented, and usually only becomes a major problem once you have a permanent post. However, trainees often become consultants in one of their training hospitals, and the leakage of personal information may start during training. Consequently, it is as well to assume that anything you reveal about yourself will become part of accumulated folk knowledge. Your home address, revealed to one patient, might as well be given to all patients. Electoral registers and Google maps mean that even revealing the general vicinity where you live may be sufficient to identify your address and enable a look at the building. The greater the patient's knowledge of you, the more difficult it is to maintain your position as a neutral figure.

Patients will often confront psychiatrists with a request for a personal disclosure:

Are you married?

Are you a parent?

Are you a Christian?

Where are you from?

This can mean that they feel you will not understand some part of their life unless you have the same beliefs or experiences as them. It is self-evident that you hardly ever meet a patient with identical beliefs and experiences as yourself. The psychiatrist's ability to understand the patient rests on factors other than similarities between them. Most psychiatrists are reluctant to make such disclosures, but try to explore with the patient why they have asked. This is a boundary issue, the message to the patient being 'In this setting, I put my personal beliefs to one side and I do not judge.'

Some psychiatrists feel that patients have a right to know some basic facts about them, and will make disclosures, but they still need to tackle the underlying issue in much the same way. Furthermore, they must carefully guard against advocacy of their political or religious beliefs, which is an abuse of power.

Finally, the doctor can offer self-disclosure as a means of powerfully illustrating a point. For example, Mrs Johnson is depressed and very troubled that she has developed checking rituals. Dr Coltrane says that this will resolve when she feels less depressed, but Mrs Johnson is not reassured. Dr Coltrane tells her that these symptoms are extremely common in the general population, and that he gets them himself when under stress. When he is very busy, he has to check the car doors and all the house locks before he can go to sleep.

However, it can easily go wrong. Mrs Johnson may feel that Dr Coltrane's symptoms are much milder than hers, and that he does not understand or that he is trivialising the problem. She may feel that the disclosure indicates that Dr Coltrane has problems, and that she should not burden him with her own. Dr Coltrane may have fallen victim to the trap of mistakenly identifying with the patient's problem. Mrs Johnson may actually have a range of undisclosed symptoms of chronic OCD. In leaping to this identification and disclosure, he has foreclosed further exploration of the symptoms.

Voluntary self-disclosure should be used sparingly and only where the doctor is certain that it is pertinent and appropriate to the patient's situation. It must not be used if the doctor is struggling with significant problems. This invites a collapse of the therapeutic relationship and even a reversal of care, where the patient feels responsible for the doctor's well-being. If in doubt, it is best not to do it at all. If one does make a disclosure, it is important to be vigilant for an alteration in the quality of the relationship.

There is a vocal minority amongst UK mental health professionals who disagree about where to place the boundaries with regard to religion and spirituality. They advocate greater integration of spirituality and psychiatric practice. A protracted controversy has ensued (Poole and Cook 2011; Poole and Higgo 2011). There is no evidence base to fall back on, and there is no compromise position that has any credibility. It remains our advice that you should exercise great caution in revealing personal beliefs, whether these are religious or political, in clinical settings. We believe that practices such as praying with patients are unethical and constitute boundary violations. Whilst others disagree, they advocate great caution. All agree that there are significant risks involved.

Physical Contact

People vary in their social use of touch. Within the dominant British culture of the twentieth century, touch indicated intimacy. Outside of this, it was confined to stiff social rituals, such as shaking hands, or special situations such as goal scoring on the football field. Even small breaches of the no-touch rule can cause significant awkwardness among older Britons. A brief lingering handshake can feel very inappropriate to a middle-aged Englishman. Other cultures, of course, follow entirely different rules. In recent times Britain has become altogether less touch averse. Younger people hug each other in a manner that appears positively promiscuous to their elders. There is still a substantial proportion of the UK population that finds the degree of ordinary social touching prevalent in parts of the USA intrusive, despite the fact that it is now commonplace for British men to greet each other with an extravagant bear-hug.

This variation means that socially tactile doctors have to restrain themselves in clinical settings, as touch can create confused communications. The implication of intimacy means that touch may be experienced by some patients as invasive. It may draw the patient into an inappropriate familiarity or dependency. It may promote an abuse of power.

There is a dilemma over the use of touch where the patient is distressed. A hand on the forearm can convey concern and can be comforting where verbal communication has, for the moment, become impossible. The vignette about the abuse of power above illustrates how ambiguity over touch can lead to major problems. Touch must be unambiguous. The contact should be brief. Protracted handholding is not therapeutically helpful under any circumstances. If you are uncertain if it will be well received or understood, it is best not to touch at all.

Patients break the no-touch taboo when disinhibited. It is not a pleasant experience to be forcibly kissed by someone who is manic. As far as possible, such advances should be repelled, and you should make it clear that your personal space must be respected. This demands reciprocation; you have to respect your patient's personal space too.

Contact Outside of the Clinical Setting

Psychiatrists will occasionally meet patients and their families away from the workplace. It is impossible to prevent. People bump into each other in the street, or the psychiatrist may come across the patient in their own occupational role. Most patients will acknowledge the doctor as an acquaintance. Some wish to act as if they do not know the psychiatrist, and this must be respected as an aspect of confidentiality. Consequently, the doctor has to await the patient's social cue before either returning a greeting or doing nothing. Some patients are more effusive. They want to update the doctor on how they are doing, or they invite a change of relationship from therapeutic to social ('Let's go for a drink!'). They may want to introduce the doctor to their friends. Mostly, such approaches are friendly and are not recognised by the patient as inappropriate. However, quite apart from the hazards for the therapeutic relationship, most of us do not want work to invade our own time. Fortunately, a courteous greeting and a determined moving on usually curtails the interaction and the patient is not offended.

Termination

Therapeutic relationships need a satisfactory conclusion. If they end abruptly, the patient can feel abandoned and rejected. Therapeutic progress can be lost. Abrupt termination of the relationship can arise in two ways. The first is where the doctor is leaving and neglects to inform the patient of this. Trainees move between posts, and they must give patients ample warning that they are going to leave. Inexperience leads trainees to underestimate their personal importance to their patients.

The second scenario arises when the therapeutic relationship has gone wrong, and the doctor withdraws in exasperation or panic. Unless there is a threat of actual violence to the doctor, abrupt termination is a self-indulgence that should be avoided. Even where withdrawal is the right outcome, as with Dr Parker and Mrs Redding, a little time is needed for the patient to understand and for the relationship to conclude.

A Personal Style

Understanding the main issues and pitfalls in managing therapeutic relationships helps the psychiatrist to find an appropriate personal clinical style. Some psychiatrists attempt to affect a dispassionate and distant clinical persona, following rigid and inflexible rules. Whilst this protects them from breaches of boundaries, it is rarely effective. The overall effect is cold and aloof, and it can cause considerable problems in establishing therapeutic relationships.

You bring your own personality into the consulting room, with its strengths and its weaknesses. Effective clinical styles are built on this foundation. There is no single correct way of doing things, and no advice as to how to conduct oneself will work for everyone all the time. Any style will have some drawbacks. Opaque and reserved psychiatrists tend to encounter transference problems. Open and demonstrative psychiatrists tend to encounter dependency problems. It is important that psychiatrists should possess a high degree of self-understanding and maintain a critical awareness of what is going on within each therapeutic relationship. They must be ready to adjust their approach according to the nature of the patient's problem, and in the light of what happens over time.

Main Points in This Chapter

1. The rules of professional behaviour establish boundaries to therapeutic relationships that must be guarded by the doctor.
2. Guarding these boundaries creates dilemmas.
3. Breaches of boundaries tend to occur insidiously, and without vigilance they can go unnoticed. Even in the absence of professional misconduct, the consequences can be damaging to the patient.
4. When cases go wrong, review sometimes reveals an unwitting boundary breach. Recognition of this can guide remedial action.
5. Rationalisation of boundary breaches invites repetition. It is a dangerous pattern.

Difficult Interviews

Not all interviews are easy to conduct. This section concerns the types of interview which inexperienced interviewers find most anxiety provoking and troublesome. One way of understanding why these interviews are difficult is that there are hard-to-reconcile differences between the professional's and the patient's agendas. Once these differences are recognised, it may be possible to fully or partially resolve them. What is quite certain is that difficult interviews can only be successful when the interviewer has a clear understanding of the patient's likely motivations and points of view.

Difficulties Relating to Psychosis

Many health professionals struggle to achieve satisfactory interviews with psychotic patients. If doctors in general are guilty of failing to see things from their patients' points of view, this is particularly true when the patient is psychotic. In everyday language, the term 'psychotic' is taken to imply that the person is totally irrational and that their viewpoint can be ignored. Psychotic patients are still sometimes treated by health professionals as if they are oblivious, only being addressed directly in order to demonstrate psychopathology (though thankfully this is far less common than it once was).

Psychosis affects all aspects of psychological functioning, but personality does not disappear during episodes of psychosis. It is possible to make contact with the person despite the disorder. Events during psychosis are part of the person's life history and they have a significant impact after recovery.

This is not to deny that it can be very difficult to understand psychotic people, though it is rarely impossible. However, you cannot expect to form useful relationships with patients with florid psychosis if you lack a basic understanding of what it feels like to be psychotic.

The term 'psychosis' embraces a wide range of mental states. There are no general statements about it that do not have significant exceptions. Acute schizophrenia is a useful example of psychosis, as it is common and it involves experiences that are hard for most people to understand. There are limitations in taking such an example. Not everything stated here holds true under all circumstances.

Acute schizophrenia involves more than a combination of delusions and hallucinations. It is a profound disorder of fundamental psychological functioning. Psychiatrists believe that the problem is one of brain dysfunction. This view was once controversial, but it is now generally accepted that something goes seriously wrong with the basic operations of the cerebral hardware. For example, there is growing evidence that acute schizophrenia is associated with cerebral inflammatory processes in a significant minority of cases. Nonetheless, psychosis occurs in the context of meaningful stresses and important situational problems. Psychotic ideas are often understandable in these terms. Although the mental state abnormalities may be due to more than a psychological reaction, the things that psychotic patients say remain meaningful (Laing 1990).

For many years, psychiatric research into schizophrenia endeavoured to identify sub-types, symptom clusters and their underlying causes. The research strategy followed a paradigm taken from general medicine. It has not been greatly successful. Underlying biological causes have proven elusive or non-specific. Recently, there is evidence that a large number of genes of small effect confer a vulnerability to schizophrenia, but the same genes are also associated with a range of other mental disorders (Kavanagh et al. 2015). We have a lot of knowledge, but much less understanding, of the nature of schizophrenia.

On the other hand, the epidemiology of the disorder is well understood, together with those factors that worsen or relieve the symptoms. Whilst treatment of the condition has improved, this is not based upon an understanding of the neurological basis of the condition. In fact, in both treatment and in potential prevention strategies, understanding of the social and psychological aspects of the disorder has been more helpful. At the time of writing, they still appear more promising to us (Poole et al. 2014). Biological research is important, but it casts little light on the subjective experience of being psychotic. Understanding the patient's experience is an important part of forming a therapeutic relationship with them.

Psychological understanding always has a foundation in observation and empathy, but it may be improved if you have access to different ways in which the person's state of mind can be understood. Clinical psychologists have done a great deal of empirical research to try to understand how schizophreniform symptoms come about, especially delusions and hallucinations. There are older models, some of which are phenomenological, and some of which are based on psychoanalysis. Over the years, we have found all three of these helpful in different ways.

There are similarities and continuities between modern psychological models and older models. There are also large gaps in all of them, even the more empirically based modern ones. It is important not to mistake any of these explanatory models for well-established hard fact. They are helpful in thinking about and understanding patients' experiences. They are of no value whatsoever in understanding how an individual might behave under a given set of circumstances. There is a body of knowledge that has some predictive power in psychosis and there are factors that are known to affect course, outcome, risk and treatment choice. These models are not part of that. Over-attachment to a particular model can have the opposite effect to that intended. Understanding can be impaired, not enhanced, and relationships with patients can be damaged, not improved.

Boxes 7.1, 7.2 and 7.3 briefly summarise some of the ideas that we have found helpful in understanding our patients suffering from schizophrenia. Other clinicians have found a range of other frameworks helpful. We make no claims for the superiority of those that we have chosen to set out here.

The experience of being psychotic does not conform closely to popular concepts of madness. The man who thinks he is Napoleon and organises the Russian campaign from his garden shed is a stereotype that does not occur in real life. People do not become lost in coherent delusional worlds; they exist in the here and now, their usual personalities and habits moving in and out of focus as they struggle to cope with their mental dysfunction and the demands of reality.

People with chronic schizophrenia can be entirely normal in their demeanour, coping well with the nuisance of hallucinations, and holding delusional beliefs that are no more important than unusual opinions. In acute psychosis, the situation is different. The disorder is pervasive and yet fluctuating. The patient is aware of the real world and is capable of responding to it, but the capability is impaired and intermittent. Rudeness, disrespect or brutality have their usual effects on a psychotic person and are rarely forgotten or forgiven when psychosis passes.

BOX 7.1 Bleuler's Model of Schizophrenia

Eugen Bleuler coined the term 'schizophrenia' over 100 years ago. According to Bleuler, the primary symptoms of the disorder were abnormal associations, autism, abnormal affect and ambivalence (sometimes called the four 'A's'). Abnormal, or loosened, associations meant that ideas did not connect in the normal logical way. At its most pronounced, this consists of 'knight's move thinking'. Autism did not refer to autistic spectrum disorder as we would now understand it, but to inward preoccupation and loss of interest in the external world. Abnormal affect referred to both unreactive (or flattened) affect and incongruous affect, usually empty giggling. Ambivalence (or 'ambitendence') refers to an intense indecisiveness and inability to form or to follow through intentions. These features are seen in 'negative' symptoms of schizophrenia, usually evident once the illness has become chronic, and in schizophreniform thought disorder.

To Bleuler, the symptoms that were later identified by Kurt Schneider as pathognomic of the condition (or 'first rank') were secondary to these more fundamental aspects. However, Schneiderian first rank symptoms are still commonly seen, but the Bleulerian four 'A's' are less evident in patients since the large mental hospitals closed. Far from being fundamental to the disorder, they may have been partly due to, or exacerbated by, the social environment that patients lived in.

BOX 7.2 Psychoanalytic Model of Schizophrenia

Some psychoanalysts regard the fundamental problem at the heart of schizophrenia to be 'psychotic turmoil'. It corresponds to the presentation of classical hebephrenic schizophrenia. This is a subtype of schizophrenia that has an early and insidious onset and is dominated by thought disorder. Thinking lacks goal direction and logical syntax is impaired. Thoughts are connected in ways that are hard for others to understand. There is an inability to distinguish core and peripheral aspects of ideas. This causes problems in the evaluation of the outside world. Whilst associations between ideas become loose, concepts become more concrete. Emotions lose coherence and become disconnected from related thoughts. The person experiences everything as confusing and changed, and their inner turmoil starts to threaten their sense of self. The sense of self has a crucial psychological function, as it allows us to understand who we are as unitary, continuous and whole persons. It allows us to understand that we have not ceased to exist whilst sleeping. It creates a boundary between ourselves and the outside world.

Eventually, living with such a mental state becomes very frightening. In the absence of coherent thought or feelings, the person is unable to distinguish what is arising from within himself and what is arising externally. Psychoanalysis, which is strong on poetic turns of phrase, describes this as the abyss of personal annihilation; falling forever and falling to pieces. The florid symptoms of schizophrenia are understood as an attempt to restore the core sense of self by redrawing the boundaries of self and arbitrarily attributing unpleasant and disturbing experience to the outside world. A coherent sense of self is restored by abandoning reality testing. Living in a threatening world is less frightening than losing oneself completely.

BOX 7.3 Experimental Psychology Model of Schizophrenia

Many clinical psychology researchers who are interested in psychosis (e.g. Bentall 2003) completely reject the validity of the concept of schizophrenia as a syndrome. Instead they focus on specific symptoms, mainly paranoid beliefs and auditory hallucinations. They link these to underlying dysfunctional ways of thinking about self and the world, in turn based upon adverse childhood experience. They stress that hallucinations and, to a lesser extent, paranoid thinking are widespread in the general population. They reject a clear distinction between 'normality and 'mental illness'.

Such a model would suggest that a child who experiences recurrent victimisation develops insecure attachment. Consequently, they use normal psychological mechanisms involved in the anticipation and avoidance of social threat at a much lower threshold than other people. As they grow older, their damaged self-esteem moves from 'bad-me' ('people mistreat me because I deserve it') to 'poor-me' ('I am being persecuted'). Acute psychosis consists of a transition between these psychological schemata, an alteration from feeling unhappy in the world to being actively persecuted by others. Similarly, hallucinations arise when the habitual negative internal speech of poor self-esteem is reframed as the negative speech of external, persecutory, others.

A Patient with Acute Schizophrenia

Gavin was 16 years old when his parents noticed that he was becoming quieter. He stopped playing football for the school team for no obvious reason. He started spending long periods in his bedroom listening to music. His school performance deteriorated, and his attendance became erratic. His parents felt that something was worrying him, perhaps his lack of a girlfriend, but even tactful questioning led to angry denials and periods of silent hostility.

Gavin certainly did not feel too good. He found it hard to concentrate and often fell into the grip of a miserable sense of confusion. Unable to make sense of what was wrong, he searched for meaning in metaphysical ideas. He became interested in philosophy and psychology, and spent hours flicking through books whilst alone in his room. Sometimes, a particular turn of phrase or a concept seemed to sum up what was wrong with the world, and he would briefly feel elated, but when he tried to explain his insights to others, the ideas would slip away from him and he was left with an empty feeling of puzzlement. Tasks, such as writing an essay, which once came easily to him, required tremendous effort. He felt uncomfortable around his friends, who seemed to be in on a joke that he could not understand. He felt most at ease when alone. It made him angry when people asked what was wrong. He did not know what was wrong, but it seemed to be related to the state of the world.

Eventually, Gavin's mother insisted on taking him to their GP. She explained his change in behaviour. Gavin said he was fine, just a bit tired. The GP asked him about drug use, which he denied. On direct questioning, he confirmed that he was worried about not having a girlfriend and about his poor academic performance. The GP felt he was suffering from an adolescent stress reaction and he said to come back if things were no better in a few months.

Three months later, things were worse. Gavin had a continuous headache and a queasy sense of apprehension. Even minor decisions took a huge effort. He stopped attending school and lay in bed trying not to think of anything. The rest of the house seemed alien and changed. He found it hard to understand what his parents were saying. He felt sure that something awful was about to happen. He was dragged back to the GP, where he was sullen and miserable. The doctor felt that he was now frankly depressed, and prescribed an antidepressant.

Although Gavin protested that there was nothing wrong with him, his mother pressed him into taking the tablets. After a few days, he seemed to be improving. He started going out again. Three days after starting the tablets, Gavin noticed that an old Pink Floyd record contained a special message for him. It implied that he had a responsibility to prevent the destruction of the planet. At first he was relieved to find a meaning in all the confusing changes that had been going on around him. He started to notice more messages, and felt that he had to visit various places he had known as a child. People were looking at him oddly. He felt that they could read his thoughts. A voice started giving him advice and instructions, sometimes friendly, sometimes threatening. Although he was frightened, life seemed meaningful and his terrible lethargy lifted.

When Gavin's parents overheard him laughing to himself in his room, they started to feel really worried. Now when they questioned him, he angrily insisted that they knew perfectly well what was happening. One evening, he stormed into the house and demanded that his parents give him the 'heart key'. He became frustrated at their inability to understand and he threw a clock through a closed window.

The following day, Gavin was lying on his bed, listening to his FM radio. He had tuned between stations and was listening to a voice that he could hear within the white noise, telling him that he would die sexually if he did not get the heart key. There was a knock at the door, and his mother walked in, followed by the GP and Dr Coltrane who was introduced as 'a specialist who has come to see you'. Gavin was angered by the sudden intrusion, especially as he needed to concentrate on the radio. He irritably ordered the threesome out of his room. He complained of their rudeness at coming in uninvited and without a prior appointment. He turned the radio up and the voice warned him not to talk to the doctors, who were trying to keep him away from the heart key.

Gavin was agitated by the turn of events. He felt torn between cooperation and withdrawal. He respected doctors, and he wanted to talk about what was happening to him. However, he did not know who Dr Coltrane was, and it was possible that he was a mind reader. The excitement of the moment set off a riot of fragmented thoughts and feelings. He had a strong urge to get out, if not through the door, then out of the window. He would like to sit down and explain, but just now he needed the chance to calm down. Dr Coltrane asked the others to leave and said that he would leave too, if Gavin insisted, but that it might be useful to talk.

The Psychiatrist's Agenda

Interviewing an acutely psychotic patient for the first time is different from an ordinary interview. Attempts to adhere rigidly to a standard format are doomed to failure. This is not to say that the systematic acquisition of information can be neglected. On the contrary, it is important to ensure that the history is comprehensive, as it is likely to be delivered in a muddled way. Information is likely to come from a range of sources. Sometimes it takes several interviews to clarify important background history. The patient may not have engaged in the interview willingly. The doctor is likely to have significant information prior to speaking to the patient.

1. When interviewing someone with acute psychosis, the psychiatrist's agenda is dominated by the need to do something. The dominance of this item represents a major problem in establishing a therapeutic relationship with the patient. It is likely that the doctor will be prepared to force action on the patient if it proves impossible to reach a safe and satisfactory plan by agreement. The psychiatrist wants to contain the risk that the patient will harm himself or somebody else. In any case, he or she is likely to feel that the patient will only deteriorate without treatment. Family, friends or police are often involved and they are likely to press hard for some form of intervention. This agenda item dominates as soon as it is clear that the patient is psychotic, and long before assessment is complete. It can be reframed as the question 'What is an appropriate intervention, and how am I going to get the patient to accept it?'

2. The psychiatrist needs to understand the overall situation. This requires sufficient background information to understand who the patient is, what effect the illness has on the patient's daily functioning and on those around them, what supports they have, and what concerns are held by those closest to the patient. Evidence of aggressive or self-harming behaviour is important, as is evidence of self-neglect. Substance misuse is significant, as it can lead to sudden alterations in behaviour, and can compound impaired judgement.

3. The psychiatrist wants to understand the patient's current mental state. This does not just mean eliciting psychopathology, but also understanding the patient's concerns and wishes. Understanding that a psychotic patient is concerned for the welfare of their cat, and that they will only go into hospital if the cat is properly cared for, can be an important component in achieving treatment on a cooperative basis. Psychopathology does matter. For example, command hallucinations or jealous delusions are associated with dangerous behaviour. However, there is much more to the psychotic patient than the sum of their symptoms.

4. An impression must be formed of the *trajectory* that the situation is following. This is not a term that is familiar from psychiatric textbooks, but it is a concept that is important to all practising psychiatrists. Trajectory includes both direction and speed. By taking all the available information together, it is possible to form an impression of how rapidly the situation is developing and whether adverse events are likely to occur. Both illness characteristics and contextual factors, such as the capacity of those coping with the situation to carry on in this role, are drawn together to assess trajectory. It is a key factor in deciding, for example, between inpatient and community treatment.

5. The psychiatrist is trying to win the patient's trust. This must not be done through trickery or dishonesty. It can be impossible to win a psychotic patient's trust. Where it can be achieved, it makes a substantial difference to the ease with which treatment proceeds and to the patient's experience of treatment.

6. If this fails, the psychiatrist wishes to have some authority in the situation. This does not correspond to being authoritarian, which tends to evoke hostility. It is helpful for the psychiatrist to be in charge in these situations in a way that would otherwise be quite inappropriate.

7. The psychiatrist wishes to behave in a way that will withstand retrospective scrutiny. A therapeutic relationship cannot be built on foundations of patronising, dismissive or bullying behaviour. The doctor may be at the start of a lengthy relationship with the patient. The doctor must later be able to justify to the patient what has been done and the manner in which he or she did it.

The Psychotic Patient's Agenda

You cannot assume that this will be incoherent. The following is a list of agenda items that patients may bring to interviews. It is not exhaustive, and an individual will not carry them all.

1. Psychotic patients often engage in an interview with a psychiatrist because they have been told to do so. They follow a pattern of deference and social convention. They have no clear idea of the purpose of the interview, and they have no positive expectations of the outcome. This is anxiety provoking. Anyone would be anxious about an interview, without an evident purpose, that has been arranged by someone else.

2. Many psychotic patients want something from the psychiatrist that is compatible with their agenda. They may simply want to unburden themselves, to talk with someone outside of the situation about the bad things that have been happening. They may want help with the situation. They are unlikely to see this in the same terms as the psychiatrist, but nonetheless, they may feel that the doctor is an appropriate person to turn to for assistance. For example, paranoid patients may seek sanctuary through hospital admission in order to escape persecutors, rather than because they feel that they are ill. They may feel depressed and suicidal and want psychiatric help with this, rather than with the psychotic symptoms that are causing them to despair.

3. Psychotic patients sometimes want something from the psychiatrist that is not compatible with the doctor's agenda. For example, patients often want the psychiatrist to support their point of view, to agree that they are not unwell when others are suggesting that they are, or to confirm that their delusional beliefs are based on reality. They can demand inappropriate interventions, such as surgery to remove a radio from their abdomen or hypnosis to reveal a hidden truth.

4. Most patients are looking for someone they can trust, because they are frightened and confused and do not know what to do. It is hard to trust anyone when you are psychotic, but doctors have an advantage in winning trust because of the special status of the medical profession.

5. Believing that there is nothing wrong with them, some patients simply want to escape the psychiatrist's attention, to get out of the interview and to be left alone. This may take the form of wanting to explain that they are fine, but it may be much more hostile than this. Young men, wary of the police in general and now taken against their will to hospital in a police van, are likely to view the psychiatrist as an arm of oppressive authority, and attempt to deal with him or her by silence or threats.

Reconciling the Agendas

It may be impossible to resolve fully the conflicts between the psychiatrist's and patient's agendas in these situations. It is usually possible to reconcile enough to establish a therapeutically useful relationship, or at least to allow such a relationship to flourish at a later time. A permanent skew can enter into the relationship, with the patient permanently viewing the psychiatrist as a benign but controlling authority figure. Sometimes the relationship contains an element of permanent active hostility, though the expression of this varies over time.

There are two elements that assist reconciliation of agendas. One is the way that the psychiatrist conducts the interview, and the other is the active process of negotiation.

Conducting the Interview

Successful interviews with psychotic patients do not require complex techniques. The main requirement is for a heightened attention to the ordinary rules of interviewing with some accommodation to the vulnerabilities and difficulties of someone who is acutely psychotic.

Psychotic patients cope badly with stimulating environments. They have particular problems with ambiguity and with distracting stimuli. Calmness and openness are helpful. Familiar social behaviour is reassuring, whilst anything suggestive of covert motives or frank trickery is alarming.

There is a need to consider the setting in which one conducts the interview. Doctors often find themselves in an environment over which they have little control, such as an accident and emergency department (A&E), the patient's home or a police station. Nonetheless, it is usually possible to take some steps to make the situation easier for the patient.

As far as possible, the interview should be conducted one-to-one and in privacy. This often means removing other people from the room. If the patient feels safer with a friend or family member present, this can be helpful, provided they are asked not to intervene (complex three-way dialogues are difficult for both the patient and the doctor). Interruptions from outside and extraneous noise are very unhelpful, and others should be asked to avoid this.

If the doctor is fearful, the patients will pick this up and become more fearful themselves. It is essential that the doctor feels safe. The interview should be unhurried, and the doctor should be firm but polite. Most patients who are psychotic are reassured by the feeling that the doctor is in control of the interview. The doctor should be as open as possible, explaining why he or she is there and what his or her concerns are. It must be clear that the doctor is listening sympathetically, neither challenging nor confirming delusional ideas. The doctor must acknowledge the patient's distress and attend to the patient's realistic concerns. The doctor is looking for common ground during the interview, identifying those items in the patient's agenda which correspond to his or her own, in order to allow a negotiation.

Negotiating with Psychotic Patients

Negotiation implies that full reconciliation of agendas is not possible. In a negotiation, some agenda items have to be abandoned by one side or the other in order to achieve a plan of action that is acceptable to both parties. If this cannot be achieved, cooperation, which is normally a prerequisite of doctor–patient relationships, will break down, temporarily or permanently. In practice either party can implement this: in the patient's case by running away, and in the doctor's case by initiating compulsory action under mental health legislation.

It is conventional to state that psychotic patients can be treated without compulsion, provided they have 'good insight'. Insight is, however, a difficult concept, hard to define and not located solely in the patient. Insight really means the degree to which the patient agrees with the doctor. 'Good insight' is the outcome of a negotiation between the doctor and the patient, aimed at finding an accommodation over what is wrong in order to work together. Insight is not a quality of the patient, but of the relationship.

The process of finding common ground is a dynamic one, with both doctor and patient playing an active role. Most patients feel that they have a problem, even if they believe it is external to them. There is little point in the doctor forcing a formulation of the problem that is totally unacceptable to the patient ('Well, actually it isn't the freemasons that are the problem. You have acute paranoid schizophrenia and you need hospitalisation'), but it is also unhelpful to collude dishonestly with delusions ('The freemasons won't be able to get you on Ward 5'). The doctor must find a position that is honest but not confrontational. For example, 'You will feel safer on Ward 5.' This bypasses the question of belief in the delusion and establishes a truthful common concern. It implies that a problem is located in the patient, laying the ground for later negotiations.

Negotiations are necessary on all kinds of issues in the continuing relationship between the doctor and the patient, and often stretch far into the future. The principles are unchanging. The most serious pitfall is dishonesty. For example, it is very tempting to suggest that a patient should come into the hospital for a few days for a rest, in the hope that this sounds so innocuous that the patient will accept it. The doctor knows that the admission is likely to last weeks, it is unlikely to be restful, and that any attempt to leave will lead to detention. The 'few days' rest' offer is unethical and causes problems later. When the patient finds he or she is unable to leave hospital, he or she is unlikely to find it easy to trust the psychiatrist again. The admitting doctor has pulled an expedient trick on the patient that has persistent adverse consequences. Promises of rapid recovery, side effect-free medication, or any other untenable undertaking, will similarly damage long-term therapeutic relationships.

Detained Patients

The detention of patients in hospital is an unavoidable reality of psychiatric practice. Without detention, significant numbers of seriously ill patients would suffer, deteriorate or die. That small minority of psychotic patients who are dangerous when unwell would commit offences and then would be imprisoned.

Most psychiatrists dislike detaining patients. They recognise that once a patient has been detained, the therapeutic relationship is forever altered, though not necessarily destroyed. The knowledge that psychiatrists have the power to detain affects relationships with patients far beyond those who actually experience detention. Treating a patient under compulsion introduces a new agenda item into the relationship between the doctor and the patient, namely the issue of control.

The psychiatrist's power over detained patients is extensive. Detention is a major event in the patient's life. However, it is a routine aspect of the psychiatrist's work. The psychiatrist is familiar with the psychiatric ward and becomes desensitised to the disturbed and disturbing aspects of this environment. Modern inpatient units are more attentive to patients' needs than mental hospitals were in the past, when patients had no rights and little ability to make complaints. Consequently, professionals tend to see detention as relatively benign, and lose sight of the nightmarish quality of the experience.

We usually think of freedom as a political issue, the right to free expression and free association. We tend not to think of more banal freedoms, which are usually only lost in the context of imprisonment. Detained patients, it can be argued, have less freedom even than a prisoner. They are held under far more ambiguous rules. The experience of being detained, coming together as it does with acute mental illness, is very frightening. The doctor may not feel powerful, but he or she is exerting extensive control over the patient. It is inevitable that the effect on the subsequent relationship is profound.

The Experience of Being Detained

Gavin was admitted from home under compulsion a few days after the psychiatrist's visit. He had initially agreed to take medication, but never did. He had come to believe that his parents were mind readers. In an argument, he threw a cup at his father, cutting his father's head.

That evening he was arguing with the voice in the radio, which was telling him that he was about to die sexually, when there was some noise outside the house. He went out to find his parents, the doctors, two social workers, two ambulance men and three policemen in earnest discussion. Panic stricken, he rushed back to his room. There was a series of shouted conversations through the locked door, with implausible reassurances followed by escalating threats of forced entry. A hastily constructed barricade of furniture proved inadequate when the police forced the door open. He was bundled down the stairs and into the ambulance in handcuffs, whilst he screamed for help and pleaded to be left alone.

The ward was institutional, despite homely touches and domestic furniture. The staff were calm and pleasant, but to Gavin it was obvious that they were part of the plot against him. He was extremely wary of them. He slept badly in a small dormitory full of strangers. Over the next few days, Gavin felt that his plight had worsened. He did not trust the staff, and the other patients were obviously mentally disturbed. He was told that if he tried to leave, he would be stopped, by force if necessary. There seemed little point in appealing for release to the same authorities that had acted against him. He was not allowed to collect his belongings from home, or to go to the local shops. He was forced to follow a routine of meal times that were rigid and against his normal pattern. He was not allowed to lie on his bed when he wanted to. He was permitted no privacy and was constantly observed by staff, even when washing.

He was given tablets which he was told would make him feel better, but they made him drowsy. His hands shook and he felt constantly restless. His mouth was dry, but he could only have a cup of tea at certain times. He observed that refusal of tablets could lead to quite brutal forced injections. He had no idea why he was being held in these conditions. There was no indication as to what he had to do in order to be released, other than to submit to the regime. He soon abandoned protest and did as he was told. The situation was quite hopeless. His spirit was broken.

Compulsory treatment was the right thing under the circumstances, but it was still oppressive. No matter how humane the regime, it is inevitable that many patients find the experience similarly unpleasant. Gavin eventually recovered and told the psychiatrist that hospital admission had been the right intervention, but the impact of this exercise of power over Gavin remained within their relationship.

Long after release from hospital, the patient is aware that defiance of the psychiatrist's advice may lead to further detention. For the relationship to be helpful to the patient, this issue needs to be an open one. The doctor must make it clear from the outset why they think that detention is appropriate, what they think is wrong and the purpose and nature of the treatment. These have to be explained in terms that the patient can understand, which will vary over time. Even if the patient disagrees with what has been done, it is possible to have a therapeutic relationship on the basis that the doctor is well intentioned. The exercise of control is most damaging when it appears arbitrary and capricious.

Some patients are reassured by being detained. When everything is frightening and out of control, it can be reassuring to return to a more child-like position where someone else takes charge and makes difficult decisions for you. Repeatedly detained patients can become quite dependent upon their psychiatrist, and you have to work within this dependency. It is not the same as the emotional dependency of the anxious outpatient, who needs to attend the clinic regularly in order to feel secure. For these more severely ill patients, the psychiatrist has a major impact on their material circumstances, not just in detaining them, but in helping them to secure benefits, housing and daytime activities. They sometimes invite a doctor who has held them unwillingly in hospital to attend major life ceremonies, such as weddings and christenings.

Dealing with Psychotic Patients Who Are Frightening

Most inexperienced doctors are uneasy when interviewing psychotic patients, but open fearfulness is unhelpful. Fear militates against careful listening and decision-making. A fearful doctor will make the patient feel worse. Fear raises the degree of emotional arousal in the interview. It creates ambiguities and a sense of insecurity that feeds patients' paranoid feelings.

Psychotic patients can be frightening even when they do not pose a threat to the doctor. The more a patient is similar to oneself, the less likely they are to invoke fear. Conversely, those types of persons who are most likely to cause apprehension in ordinary life seem most frightening when mentally disturbed. Differences in ethnicity and class can contribute to a fearfulness that is not related to any immediate realistic threat. You need to be aware that fear may be more related to prejudice than to objective risk.

Unpredictability is frightening. Experienced psychiatrists are more comfortable than trainees in the presence of psychotic patients. Their behaviour is more predictable to doctors with a good understanding of psychotic mental states. People who are psychotic interact differently from other people. Their emotional rapport and body language are wrong, and this creates unease. They may be difficult to converse with. Their suspiciousness or perplexity is uncomfortable for other people. Above all, states of over-arousal are intensely unsettling for the doctor. The patient is restless, tense, sweaty and hypervigilant; the condition signals danger.

People who are psychotic can be aggressive or violent. In general, psychotic patients become aggressive either because they are frightened or because they are frustrated. The major exceptions to this are manic patients who in a state of elation and excitement may become indiscriminately aggressive as an intrinsic part of the mood abnormality.

Needless to say, the process of psychiatric assessment offers ample opportunity for a psychotic patient to become frightened or frustrated. Most patients who are going to be aggressive show clear signs of this by the time the psychiatrist arrives. You are often confronted by a very angry person at the beginning of the interview. It is unusual for aggression to arise unexpectedly in the course of an interview. The key to calming such patients is to be calm yourself. To achieve this, you have to ensure that the degree of personal danger is minimal. You should refuse to conduct the interview until this is achieved. This insistence can create an uncomfortable impression of cowardice, especially within the macho culture of hospital medicine. It may mean refusing to see a patient who is at risk at home until others are available to attend with you. Failure to achieve this does the patient a disservice. The psychiatrist's interview and assessment are likely to have major consequences. They cannot be carried out appropriately by a doctor who is desperate to get away from the patient. The issue of safety is discussed in greater depth in Chapter 19.

Main Points in This Chapter

1. Interviews with patients suffering from acute psychosis require a different technique to other clinical interviews. The basic principles of the interaction and relationship are otherwise unchanged.
2. Psychosis can be understood. The patient's individual wishes and concerns remain meaningful, despite the mental state abnormality.
3. Psychiatric intervention may curtail the patient's freedom and autonomy. This damages the therapeutic relationship. The damage is minimised by retaining an awareness of how one's actions are received, and by engaging in a process of honest negotiation.
4. Psychotic patients can be frightening irrespective of the realistic danger. Measures that secure the doctor's safety facilitate a successful interview and serve the patient's best interests.
5. A mark of truly expert psychiatrists is their ability to converse with psychotic patients in a relaxed and normal way. To achieve this one needs a good comprehension of the subjective experiences of your patients.
6. These interviews are difficult for doctors but they are considerably more difficult for patients.

Unpopular Patients

Every psychiatrist could provide a personal list of the types of patients they find problematic to treat. Such a list would be largely idiosyncratic and based on the psychiatrist's personality. Some psychiatrists like treating patients with eating disorders; others find such patients difficult and frustrating. Some experience people with alcohol problems as self-indulgent and irritating whilst others enjoy treating them, and so on. This reflects variations of interest and aptitude which are unavoidable. The positive aspect of this is that it leads to special expertise in treating specific disorders. This chapter is not concerned with these preferences.

Some types of patients have problems that create difficulties for most psychiatrists, in that it is difficult to form a useful therapeutic relationship with them. These individuals are sometimes referred to by doctors as 'heart sink patients'. The terminology is revealing, as it implies that the difficulty is at least in part related to the doctor's emotional response. 'Heart sink' implies that they induce a sense of helplessness and frustration. It would be unrealistic to deny that we all experience this with some patients from time to time. The majority of patients who habitually behave in ways that psychiatrists find difficult also have a sense of frustrated helplessness. Doctor and patient mirror each other's feelings.

Dysfunctional doctor–patient interactions are characterised by a failure to find an accommodation between the doctor's and the patient's agendas. These patients often carry agenda items that they cannot or will not make explicit, but which are implicit in their behaviour. They cannot always be helped. An understanding of the dysfunctional therapeutic dynamic at least eases the doctor's sense of despair.

As in many dysfunctional situations in life, both parties in these unhappy clinical situations repetitively attempt to deploy strategies that have already failed. The trick is to find new, more adaptive strategies. Sometimes, the process of thinking about the problem differently will reveal a way forward to a more helpful interaction.

'Somatisers'

This commonly used term does not precisely correspond to 'those patients suffering from somatisation disorder'. 'Somatiser' is informal jargon that has a pejorative connotation. It refers to people who experience emotional distress as physical symptoms, or believe that their problem is wholly due to physical disease, when the doctor believes it is (at least in part) psychological in origin.

The patient commonly arrives at the psychiatrist's office determined to prove that the condition is organic. They attend in angry submission to another doctor's insistence that they should have a psychiatric assessment. The patient may be worried that physical illness is going untreated. Even before the patient is seen the psychiatrist anticipates trying to persuade the patient that he or she is wrong. The doctor and the patient have agenda items diametrically opposed to each other. It is hardly surprising that such interviews are uncomfortable and frequently unproductive. This is one subtype of rhetorical interview (see Chapter 16).

The behaviour of somatising patients suggests that they believe that physical distress is more authentic than emotional distress. They seem to feel that they can only be cared for if they are physically unwell. This is a *meta-agenda* that determines other specific agenda items, such as the search for an organic diagnosis. It is covert, hidden from the explicit content of the interview, and outside of the patient's immediate awareness. Such beliefs are sometimes culturally determined, and only cause problems where the doctor is from a different culture. Sometimes these beliefs have arisen developmentally in response to early emotional experience. In either case, such deep-seated attitudes are unlikely to change just because a psychiatrist says they are wrong. On the contrary, trying to persuade the patient that they are wrong subverts the relationship towards the anti-therapeutic. Doctor and patient can become locked in a dysfunctional relationship that is fed and sustained by their mutual inability to change the other's mind.

In assessing 'somatisers', it is best to adopt a position of neutrality with respect to the nature of their problem. This can be made explicit at the outset with a statement to the effect 'I don't know what's wrong with you. Tell me the story from your point of view.' Without this, the doctor and the patient rapidly become locked in conflict. Unless there is a statement to the contrary at the outset, the patient will assume that the doctor has an opposite view to them, and act out their side of the conflict.

Clinical scepticism is a quality that protects psychiatrists against making mistakes. It is an attitude that insists on evidence and acknowledges uncertainty. It demands that you critically evaluate everything you are told, not in a spirit of cynicism, but in the recognition that human beings get things wrong. This includes yourself and other health professionals. In treating somatisers, clinical scepticism demands a neutral position, because sometimes the patient is right. Doctors have a marked tendency to think that a problem is psychological if investigations prove negative. The diagnosis 'psychological problem' is a residual category, that which is left when other possibilities have been excluded. The psychiatrist, however, is looking for positive evidence, a plausible psychological formulation of the problem. In the absence of this, the problem may well be organic. In the fullness of time, an underlying organic problem sometimes becomes evident. A proportion of patients sent to psychiatrists with vague and allegedly psychogenic neurological symptoms turn out to have multiple sclerosis.

Most somatising patients have a combination of organic and functional problems. Patients with chronic low back pain often become very miserable because of pain and disability. There is no demonstrable back pathology and they are obviously depressed. It is often implied or frankly stated that there is nothing wrong with their back and that the problem is psychological. Not surprisingly, the implication that the problem is imaginary tends to make them angry and despairing. It seems unlikely that pain can be conjured in the total absence of a painful sensory stimulus. It is perfectly possible to sustain a soft-tissue back injury leading to muscle spasm, which hurts a lot. Soft-tissue injuries and muscle spasm do not show on MRI scans. Efforts to avoid muscle spasm create postural stresses leading to further soft-tissue damage and more muscle spasm. Depression and anxiety lead to a lowering of the pain threshold.

The psychiatrist's neutrality over organicity can allow some patients to accept this type of mixed physical and psychological explanation, which then allows a useful therapeutic relationship to develop. However, there is not always such a plausible explanation available, and some patients are too entrenched in their conflict with the medical profession to concede even this degree of psychological causation. The psychiatrist's neutrality can allow a reframing of the problem under these circumstances. For example:

I can't do anything about your symptoms, because I don't understand what's causing them, but if you felt less tense about it all, you'd probably cope with the symptoms better.

These physical symptoms are outside of my expertise, but the problems between you and the doctors aren't helping at all. Maybe we can do something about that.

This type of approach works with a significant proportion of somatisers. There are treatment strategies that are effective, but they are beyond the scope of this book. In order to deploy them, you must first form a cooperative relationship with the patient.

Patients Who Will Not Acknowledge That They Have Recovered

This is a problem that arises late in the therapeutic relationship. The doctor thinks the patient is better, but the patient will not agree. The problem can arise in a number of different ways and for a number of different reasons:

- Dependency difficulties, as in the case of Mrs Redding, described in Chapter 6. Some of these patients will state that they are well, but that they are fearful of relapse. They want continued contact in order to feel secure. The conflict in agendas here is that the doctor feels they have fully recovered, whilst the patient feels damaged by having been unwell. For them, the loss of symptoms does not equate with recovery.

- Seeking perfection: Some patients present new problems every time discharge seems imminent. A proportion of patients in the 'well but dependent' group will resist discharge in this way, but there can be different factors at play. Some patients have not shared the objective of simple symptom resolution from the beginning. They are seeking a more thorough improvement in themselves, an unrealistic hope of becoming more content with life and free of problems.

- Covert motivations for continued attendance: These include support for continuation of benefits, rehousing, early retirement on medical grounds or the avoidance of punishment by the criminal justice system (see also Chapter 16).

- There is an increasing problem in some 'recovery-orientated' services in the UK, whereby clinicians are expected to discharge patients after very short contact, and before symptoms have fully resolved. Some patients are alarmed by this, especially if they lack faith in their GP's ability to satisfactorily complete treatment.

These problems turn on a single theme. The doctor and the patient have different objectives for treatment. The seekers of perfection have unrealistic expectations. The patients who find that the fact of psychiatric attendance resolves non-psychiatric problems are using the relationship inappropriately from the doctor's point of view, though not from theirs. It is hardly surprising that people struggling to survive on the margins of society will exploit any advantage they can find. The patient who resists early discharge is responding to a mismatch in expectations of specialist treatment that arises out of rapid change in service models rather than anything unusual about the patient themselves.

As with somatisers, there can be a meta-agenda behind the more obvious conflict. These patients bring to the interaction a model of doctor–patient relationship that is radically different to the psychiatrist's. For example, the role of care-giver is, for the doctor, a temporary state, with an objective (recovery) that creates a limit to the relationship. For some patients, however, being in a cared-for relationship is an end in itself. The relationship meets needs that are not otherwise satisfied. The therapeutic relationship does not facilitate change; it only solves a problem in the here and now, and therefore there is an expectation that it should continue. In contrast to this, some patients have such a low expectation of being helped by professionals that they see the doctor as someone who must necessarily be manipulated if they are to get anything worthwhile from the relationship. For some patients, early discharge can evoke strong feelings of apprehension about the likely success of treatment, and may undermine therapeutic hopefulness.

Clarity at the outset with regard to the expected length and outcome of treatment helps to avoid this kind of difficulty, but the psychiatrist is still faced with some patients who have to be discharged more or less unwillingly. The trauma of forced discharge is eased if it is possible to identify, with the patient, the nature of the problem. Sometimes, the patient is right, and discharge is premature. Psychiatrists then have a choice between doing as they are told by their managers or doing what they believe to be right.

Patients Who Lie

Truthfulness is an elusive quality, which has more to do with intention than veracity. Very few of us are capable of complete openness even momentarily, and certainly not all the time. It is the intention to mislead that sets lying apart. Psychiatrists must be attentive to the possibility of lying. The attitude of unconditional positive regard, which is a tool of the trade, can make psychiatrists appear gullible. This is certainly preferable to the appearance of being a doubting inquisitor. It is clinical scepticism that protects psychiatrists from being misled. Clinical scepticism demands answers to questions such as: *Does this story make sense? Do the dates of events leave major gaps unaccounted for?* and *Is the patient's account consistent with other accounts?* These questions can raise the possibility that the patient is lying.

Psychiatrists cannot allow themselves to be outraged by lying. Untruthfulness may not be deliberate. It may arise because the truth involves a sensitive secret. The process of teasing out the reasons for the untruth, and the significance of the truth, are grist to the mill in helping the patient. There is a large group of patients who complain of hearing voices without displaying other psychotic symptoms. It is often said that they are 'putting it on'. Not everyone who hears voices is psychotic, and it is wrong to assume that they are lying. Within this group, there are some individuals who go on to develop a psychosis.

Patients who deliberately and determinedly lie carry a meta-agenda, which is similar to that carried by patients who wish to stay in follow-up for manipulative ends. They feel impotent. They do not believe that they will be accepted or helped if they reveal themselves as they really are. They fear that they will be rejected, or believe that they must manipulate and control other people in order to get anything from them.

Confronting patients when you are sure or almost sure that they are lying is not easy, as open disbelief compromises the doctor's neutrality and unconditional positive regard. Blunt confrontation will lead the patient to withdraw from treatment, or to the replacement of the first lie with a second lie. Untruths can be disentangled without a direct accusation. Puzzlement at inconsistencies (the 'Colombo' posture), and a refusal to be deflected from understanding these, will often eventually lead to the truth. Sometimes, the patient is so resistant that there is no alternative to stating that you feel that they are not being entirely truthful. This cannot be executed as a hostile confrontation. A constructive confrontation requires a much more neutral form of interaction, despite its intrinsically accusatory content. This takes a little practice to get right.

Some patients tell really big lies. Sometimes these are easily detected. False accounts tend to be dramatic and therefore implausible ('My whole family died in an air crash last week') or inconsistent with the verifiable facts. Full-time malingerers, for example patients with Munchausen syndrome, are few in number, but they get around a lot, and most psychiatrists get to see them from time to time. A few of them become very accomplished at their art, and there is little that the psychiatrist can do to avoid being misled by them. These pathological liars are almost impossible to work with. They usually flee on being caught out, but some just invent another elaborate story.

Patients Who Persistently Complain

These days, complaints against doctors and medical services are encouraged, and rightly so. The failings of professionals can have a serious impact upon their patients. However, there is a small group of patients who are habitual users of complaints systems. Their persistent complaints about their treatment can reflect a problem with them, rather than with the professional.

These patients are often referred after they have fallen out with their previous psychiatrist. They ask for a change of doctor, or the previous psychiatrist has had enough and has discharged them. Although they may mention doubts as to your usefulness at first meeting, they more often state an expectation that you will prove more satisfactory than the previous doctor. They often express their satisfaction with the first interview. Before long, they complain about you. Looking at the pattern of their relationship with mental health services as a whole, it can appear that complaint is the point of the exercise.

The complaints tend to be about minutiae or the intangible: that your manner is wrong; that you are too critical or lack interest in them; that you are not seeing them often enough or for long enough. Sometimes there is a dispute over the technical aspects of treatment: that you have the diagnosis wrong (*'I've been reading ICD 10. I haven't got a paranoid personality disorder, I've got an obsessional personality disorder'*); that you failed to warn about a rare side effect that has now had an implausibly devastating effect on the patient's life; or that you have misconstrued a part of the history to a third party.

One way of understanding these patients is that they have a profound belief that no one cares about them and that they are helpless. They do not believe that they can influence relationships and they do not expect that anyone will listen or truly try to help them. They feel alone and neglected, and the complaints are the angry consequence of this. Their unhappiness is experienced as being autonomous, beyond their control and unrelated to their circumstances. Even when they express initial scepticism about the doctor, they have an implicit expectation that somewhere there is an ideal psychiatrist who can put things right for them. The new doctor rapidly fails against this expectation, and the complaints resume. The doctor becomes irritated or rejects them, confirming their beliefs about themselves and sustaining the cycle. Complaints and complaints systems create an opportunity to bring the existential unfairness of their lives to the attention of a wider audience.

In order to help these patients it is essential to break the pattern of movement between doctors. A further change solves your problem, but it does nothing for the patient or for your colleagues. A refusal to raise expectations may be useful, by stating at the start that you cannot promise to be any more helpful than the doctors that the patient has seen in the past. Sometimes a time limit for involvement leads to a negotiation over what might be realistically achieved in that time. A time limit avoids an indefinite struggle if it does not work out. Suggesting that realistically you are probably the last psychiatrist in the line can have a similar effect. All of this is easy when the pattern is long established, but a similar strategy can be employed when a pattern of complaint emerges after treatment has started. In all of this, one has to bear in mind the boy who cried wolf; even habitual complainers can have a good reason for complaint.

It may be possible to help these patients to achieve a more realistic understanding of their problems and to move on from the position of querulous helplessness; but not always.

Patients Who Threaten the Doctor

Patients become threatening because they feel impotent within the relationship. They usually want something from the doctor that he or she is not prepared to give. This can include admission to hospital, or prescriptions of abusable drugs, or the provision of misleading information to another agency. Some patients threaten the doctor with violence, and many threaten to harm themselves or someone else, unless some unreasonable demand is met. These latter threats have a considerable impact in a world where psychiatrists are increasingly in fear of being held accountable for their patients' behaviour.

Threats of personal violence cannot be tolerated from patients who are not psychotic. If threats are persistent or acted upon, the police should always be involved. Aggressive people do not become less so if their actions are treated as inconsequential. Some patients persecute doctors, for example in the form of letters, emails or phone calls. Under these circumstances it is essential to inform your employers and take legal action promptly. The lack of a response to such activities can frustrate an ex-patient with a grudge and lead to an escalation of the harassment. Fortunately this occurs very rarely, but when it does you must protect yourself from it at an early stage.

Patients who threaten to harm themselves or other people are a difficult problem. Although many such patients are not mentally ill, some are. The problems they pose cannot be separated from issues of risk assessment. These are explored in Chapter 19.

A Difficult Interview

Dr Lee was the duty psychiatrist on a 12-hour shift in a busy inner city emergency department. In the course of a particular evening, he assessed four patients. Two patients had to be admitted to hospital, which involved him in lengthy and frustrating telephone negotiations in order to find available inpatient beds. He finally took a break for a snack and a cup of tea at 2.30 a.m., six and a half hours through the shift. He was about to sit down to eat when he was called to assess yet another patient.

On arrival back in the emergency department, he was asked to see Mr Cox. Mr Cox turned out to be an angry 26-year-old man who was complaining of auditory hallucinations. He was demanding to be admitted to hospital. In the course of assessment, it emerged that he was living in a rough bed-and-breakfast hotel, and that he was a heavy drinker. He was in conflict with another resident, and was short of money. It seemed likely to Dr Lee that he was concealing other factors relevant to his wish to be admitted.

Dr Lee could find no evidence that Mr Cox was seriously mentally ill. It was possible that he had alcoholic hallucinosis, but the complaints of hallucinations were vague and unconvincing. There were no other symptoms. It seemed quite clear that Mr Cox was at the end of his tether and saw admission to hospital as an available method of resolving his immediate problems.

Dr Lee was also a 26-year-old man at the end of his tether. He was hungry, thirsty and tired, and he was angered that he had to deal with an awkward patient who was not psychiatrically unwell. As the interview proceeded, the doctor and the patient became increasingly irritable with each other. Mr Cox was in difficulty. He did not know how to solve his problems, and his plan to become a psychiatric inpatient was not proceeding as he had hoped. Dr Lee was also in difficulty. If he tried to admit the patient, there would be conflict with other mental health professionals. Even if he succeeded, he would be criticised the next day for the inappropriate use of a scarce resource. If he turned the patient away there might be unpleasantness.

The doctor and the patient were locked in a dysfunctional interaction, where their immediate problems mirrored each other. These situations are common, and the only way out of them is to recognise the nature of the dysfunction, which is that doctor and patient have a lot in common, but no common ground.

Dr Lee found a way forward. He pointed out that he was feeling tired and irritable, and that Mr Cox was probably feeling the same way. The interview was going nowhere because they had become locked in a struggle where neither could give way. There was no possibility of admitting Mr Cox. This was outside of his control. In any case, lying low in hospital would not make a blind bit of difference to Mr Cox's problems. They would be the same or worse on discharge. He acknowledged that Mr Cox had real and pressing difficulties, and discussed less immediate interventions that might ease Mr Cox's difficulties. The doctor and the patient were released from their conflict, and the next morning Dr Lee referred Mr Cox to a voluntary sector alcohol counselling service.

Such strategies do not always work. However, by offering the patient an alternative way forward the doctor at least feels less helpless and angry. This can, in turn, improve the dynamic with the patient.

This chapter has not attempted to exhaustively list all types of difficult interviews and unpopular patients. We have drawn out some themes that we find useful in dealing with difficult interviews. The main principles are robust over a wide range of problems. If they are observed, dysfunctional interactions can be avoided some of the time. Chapter 16 considers some situations that are widely regarded as creating impossible problems for the psychiatrist.

Main Points in This Chapter

1. In situations where the psychiatrist finds the patient difficult, there is usually a conflict between the doctor's and the patient's agendas.
2. Sometimes this has its origins in deep-seated attitudes and beliefs of the patient. We have called this the meta-agenda. It is often outside of the patient's awareness, but it determines more explicit agenda items.
3. Patients who behave in ways that doctors find difficult often do so because they feel helpless in the relationship. The doctor may feel the same.
4. If the psychiatrist attempts to force his or her agenda on the patient, the relationship will fail. It is better to search for a strategy that will establish common ground.
5. Setting limits, by being explicit about the length and objectives of treatment, and by establishing rules of conduct, is always helpful.
6. These patients are not necessarily impossible to help.

Psychiatry is an applied science. As such, objectivity is one of its central values and strengths. Objectivity is not easily achieved, as the psychiatrist is far from neutral. This section is concerned with the impact of the mental health professional's personal characteristics as an active factor affecting interviews and assessment. This involves understanding how cultural difference, ideology and personality can affect the evaluation of, and the relationship with, the patient. We all use our personalities and other individual characteristics as a clinical tool, but to do so we need to develop self-awareness.

<table>
<tr><td>Chapter
9</td><td># Values and Beliefs</td></tr>
</table>

In Chapter 6 we explored some problems and dilemmas that can arise within interactions between psychiatrists and patients. Issues such as dependency are part of the process of the therapeutic relationship. Here, we examine the impact of the professional's own values and beliefs upon the relationship.

Everyone has their own idiosyncratic set of values and beliefs, but psychiatry itself contains values, determined by the social context from which it arises. No degree of abstraction can rid any science of intrinsic values. Absolute objectivity, in the sense of God-like detachment, is impossible. This is not to deny that there are objective realities and truths that exist independently of observers, but the truth is often complex. In psychiatry, we can only observe and explain behaviours incompletely, and frequently there are several competing partial explanations. This is no justification for abandoning the aim of objectivity. Objectivity can only be achieved in the light of an understanding of our own values and beliefs. Without this, values and beliefs interfere in our clinical judgement.

Broadly speaking, values and beliefs operate at three distinct levels.

Firstly, there are the values of the British medical profession. There are explicit, codified rules, set out as guidance by regulatory bodies, but there is also a more diverse, informal, set of shared ideas that constitute the medical subculture. Within this, there is a specifically psychiatric subculture.

Secondly, there is the individual's personal belief system, an explicit personal ideology that develops out of educational, class, family, religious and political backgrounds.

Finally, elements of personality shape implicit values, which may not be fully within our awareness. These can make particular subjects or types of patients easier or more troublesome to deal with.

Medical Values

From the time of Hippocrates onwards there has been a perceived need to set out a code of values for doctors. The formal values of British medicine were first set out by the General Medical Council (GMC) when it was formed in the nineteenth century. These values are generally liberal and rationalist, being broadly based upon the ideas of the Enlightenment. The code changes with time. For example, medical attitudes to termination of pregnancy have dramatically altered. The values behind the code arise through consensus. They are determined in part by leaders of the profession, in part by demands of the public and in part by governmental policy-makers. Although appraisal, revalidation, licensing and disciplinary action have become controversial issues for doctors, there seems to be a surprisingly high degree of agreement about the values in the code itself. Criticism of organised medicine is usually based on allegations that the profession does not adhere to its code at all times. The current formal code is set out in Box 9.1 (General Medical Council 2013).

The subcultures of medicine influence the formal code, but they can conflict with it and with each other. Significant groups of doctors hold values that, under some circumstances,

---

BOX 9.1 The Duties of a Doctor Registered with the General Medical Council (GMC 2013)

Patients must be able to trust doctors with their lives and health. To justify that trust you must show respect for human life and make sure your practice meets the standards expected of you in four domains.

Knowledge, Skills and Performance

- Make the care of your patient your first concern.
- Provide a good standard of practice and care.
  - Keep your professional knowledge and skills up to date.
  - Recognise and work within the limits of your competence.

Safety and Quality

- Take prompt action if you think that patient safety, dignity or comfort is being compromised.
- Protect and promote the health of patients and the public.

Communication, Partnership and Teamwork

- Treat patients as individuals and respect their dignity.
  - Treat patients politely and considerately.
  - Respect patients' right to confidentiality.

- Work in partnership with patients.
  - Listen to, and respond to, their concerns and preferences.
  - Give patients the information they want or need in a way they can understand.
  - Respect patients' right to reach decisions with you about their treatment and care.
  - Support patients in caring for themselves to improve and maintain their health.

- Work with colleagues in the ways that best serve patients' interests.

Maintaining Trust

- Be honest and open and act with integrity.
- Never discriminate unfairly against patients or colleagues.
- Never abuse your patients' trust in you or the public's trust in the profession.

You are personally accountable for your professional practice and must always be prepared to justify your decisions and actions.

are deviant and obstructive with regard to getting the job done. For example, there is intolerance in a proportion of the profession towards patients whom they regard as morally culpable for their own ill health. This can be directed at those with substance misuse problems, people who recurrently lacerate themselves, smokers with emphysema and so on. The problem with this attitude is not just that it is in conflict with the expectations of the formal code. Taking a position of moral condemnation makes it more difficult to form relationships with such patients, to influence their behaviour and to help them to stop harming themselves.

Subcultural values do not belong to individuals. They are group phenomena. Consequently, well-meaning and otherwise highly competent individuals can hold values that are unhelpful or deviant. Deviant values tend to arise in groups that are inward-looking and isolated. This does not require geographical isolation. It can occur in tight-knit groups who work within larger organisations, such as general hospitals.

A very agitated 28-year-old woman burst into an emergency department one evening, demanding a brain scan. She was manic and had a delusion that she had a brain tumour. She was seen by an emergency department doctor, who tried to explain that a scan was not indicated. The patient rapidly became frustrated, and suddenly assaulted the doctor. He restrained her with the assistance of nursing staff, but, in the struggle, the patient bit him, breaking his skin. The patient was admitted to the psychiatric unit under legal compulsion.

Later that night, the emergency department doctor contacted the duty psychiatrist, asking that the patient be tested for HIV and hepatitis, so that he could find out whether he needed prophylaxis or not. The duty psychiatrist explained that the patient lacked mental capacity to consent to the tests, but in any case she was refusing all investigations. The casualty officer said that in the emergency department they took the view that patients who chose to assault doctors waived their rights. They had tested patients without consent under these circumstances in the past.

Unable to reach agreement, the doctors handed the matter over to their consultants. The emergency department consultant also pressed for the patient to be tested without consent, but the consultant psychiatrist was not prepared to allow this. The conflict was resolved with the discovery of specific guidance on the GMC website, which stated that, to take blood or to carry out tests without consent was both unlawful and unethical.

Variations in subcultural values between different parts of the profession are not necessarily a bad thing. For example, the degree of interpersonal engagement with patients that is prevalent amongst psychiatrists would be inappropriate in a surgeon. Psychiatrists are often openly distressed when their patients die, and it is a shared subcultural value that this is appropriate. The same attitude would be very destructive in any branch of hospital medicine where death is a daily occurrence.

One of the strengths of medicine is that it does have an explicit code. This allows subcultural values to be measured for compatibility with society's expectations. This can occur only if you stay in touch with a wider body of opinion and debate. If you do not refer back to first principles, expedient solutions to tricky problems are likely to lead to trouble.

Personal Ideology

Similar considerations apply to personal values and beliefs. Some people work in psychiatry because of deeply held personal beliefs, for example a religious faith or a political commitment to the disadvantaged. For these professionals, there is no separation between their private values and their professional work. There is nothing wrong with this. However, these strong convictions can become a serious problem where professionals lack self-awareness or are so convinced of their own belief system that they are prepared to proselytise, or otherwise force their ideas upon patients.

Most psychiatrists have to bite their tongue from time to time. They have to put their own values to one side in the course of their work and decline to express strongly held views. However, this is not sufficient in itself to protect them from acting on their values. The trouble with deeply held beliefs is that people tend to experience them as universal truths. It takes a degree of self-discipline to monitor one's own behaviour and to ensure that decisions are not inappropriately affected by personal beliefs.

A GP referred a 30-year-old woman suffering from anxiety related to pregnancy. On assessment, it emerged that the woman was pregnant by a neighbour. Her husband knew nothing about this, and she was desperate to terminate the pregnancy within the legal time limit. She had approached her GP, who, as a first step, had referred her to a 'pregnancy counsellor'. The counsellor turned out to be the GP's wife. Over a number of interviews, she had shown the patient photographs of foetuses, in order to help the patient to consider other options. On completion of counselling, she told her GP that she still wanted an abortion. He then explained that his religious beliefs prevented him from cooperating with any termination of a pregnancy, but that he was willing to send her for a psychiatric opinion.

The GP had the right to avoid actions that conflicted with his religious beliefs. He did not have the right to covertly impose his beliefs on the patient. His beliefs were affecting his professional behaviour, and he should have made this clear at the outset. He should have made it possible for the patient to see a different practitioner, no matter how wrong he felt that the outcome would be.

More subtle expressions of belief can also be damaging. For example, some people who do not recognise the legitimacy of the state of Israel refer to the geographical location as Palestine. However, to refer to Israel as Palestine to a Jewish patient is almost certain to raise an apprehension in the patient's mind about the doctor's attitude to Jews. Irrespective of the political arguments, to use such terminology is self-indulgent and abusive, as it serves the doctor's needs, not the patient's.

Strong convictions can lead to disapproval of some types of lifestyle. There are doctors who, if given the choice, would rather have nothing to do with racists or paedophiles. Such disapproval may be understandable, but it cannot be indulged. As a doctor, you either have to be prepared to treat everybody in the same way, or not to practise at all. There is a campaign in the UK against so-called 'intolerant secularisation'. The campaigners are funded by American fundamentalist Christian groups, and amongst their aims there is an aspiration to discriminate against homosexual patients. The UK regulatory bodies have been steadfastly unsympathetic to their cause, in keeping with prevalent attitudes in the general public and the profession.

We all have ideas about how people should live, and these values can intrude into a wide range of clinical situations. The difference between a clinical judgement and a personal value can be quite ambiguous. For example, many psychiatrists, including us, believe that experiencing yourself as a helpless victim is bad for your mental health. Many doctors also abhor the compensation culture that has developed in the UK, not least because it has increased medical negligence litigation. Medical defence insurance premiums have risen correspondingly. In discouraging a patient from engaging in a medical negligence claim against another doctor, is the psychiatrist protecting the patient from the victim role, or imposing his or her own values? There is not a simple answer to the question, but it is important that psychiatrists should ask themselves such questions.

All of these examples concern beliefs and values that are explicit. They are conscious and they have a rationale. One could argue their merits. Not all values and beliefs are like this.

Implicit Values

There are some beliefs and values that are so deep-seated that we are hardly aware of them. They are rooted in our personality attributes and implicit social attitudes. They cause problems through the intermediary of feelings of embarrassment or hostility towards patients.

For example, there is a social taboo against explicit discussion of sexuality with people of the opposite sex, and a further taboo against older people acknowledging that they are sexually active.

Mrs Thompson, a 47-year-old woman, has been referred by her GP. She sees Dr Nichol, a 26-year-old psychiatric trainee. On assessment, he finds that she is depressed. She makes a good recovery on a selective serotonin reuptake inhibitor (SSRI) antidepressant. At a follow-up appointment, she wishes to discontinue the medication because of side effects. Dr Nichol asks what side effects are bothering her. Mrs Thompson says that although the tablets have helped, she can no longer achieve orgasm and this has become a real problem.

Dr Nichol is acutely embarrassed. He does not want to discuss intimate details of the patient's sexual life. He is worried that any interest may appear prurient. He is very uneasy about discussing these matters with a much older woman.

Mrs Thompson has come to the interview expecting to discuss her sexual life. There was little point in raising the issue otherwise. Dr Nichol should explore the problem a little more before coming to a decision with the patient about what to do. The only obstruction to doing this is Dr Nichol's own values and inhibitions. He cannot stop himself from being uncomfortable by an act of will. Even after years of experience, some doctors remain uneasy talking with their patients about sexual matters. There is no easy way around this. Sexual issues have to be discussed, whether the doctor is comfortable with it or not. If Dr Nichol acknowledges to himself that the problem is his, he stands a better chance of overcoming the difficulty. All forms of avoidance heighten anxiety; overcoming avoidance lessens it. Skirting around difficult subjects does not help much. Grasping the nettle and forcing oneself to break the taboo tends to work a lot better.

Values and beliefs can strongly colour expectations of patients with particular types of problems. Many doctors have very negative ideas about substance misusers, whom they characterise as self-pitying, dishonest, manipulative and potentially aggressive. The doctor does not have to express such ideas for them to be a problem. They are bound to make him uncomfortable when interviewing substance misusers. He is hardly likely to be very helpful to these patients. On the other hand, some doctors feel no hostility towards substance misusers, but have a very narrow understanding of substance misusing lifestyles. This makes it difficult to obtain a substance misuse history, and ignorance can lead to an underestimation of the range of health problems caused by substance misuse. Alternatively, it can lead to the doctor inappropriately attributing all the patient's problems to substance misuse, thus missing other treatable conditions.

It is impossible to practise psychiatry effectively unless you have the capacity to understand lifestyles different from your own. For example, drugs are everywhere and all psychiatrists treat drug users. The only way of learning about the subject is either to immerse yourself in drug taking (a course that we do not recommend), or to learn from your patients. Fixed stereotypes stand in the way of hearing what patients tell you. Prejudices can only be challenged if you acknowledge that you have them.

Paedophiles

If there is one group of people who really test psychiatrists' ability to rise above their personal values, it is paedophiles. Although many mental health professionals distance themselves from modern witch-hunts and vigilante actions against paedophiles, in general they feel no more sympathy towards child-sex offenders than anyone else does. Paedophiles are the most vilified group in modern society, and most psychiatrists are far from neutral in their attitude towards them. This is exacerbated by a fear that attempts to understand a paedophile might lead to accusations of being an apologist for them. The extent of the opprobrium that paedophiles attract makes this a frightening prospect.

It is not unusual for paedophiles to be referred to general psychiatrists. They sometimes have a suicidal crisis in the face of legal action. Sometimes they seek support for their claims that they are innocent victims of malicious accusations. Sometimes paedophiles develop mental illnesses that have little or nothing to do with their sexual behaviour. No one likes paedophilic sex offenders. They rarely like each other. They retain the loyalty of friends and family only by convincing them that they are innocent. Anyone who deals with paedophiles regularly knows that they are plausible liars. This creates a further dilemma, as some people accused of paedophilic offences are innocent, and become depressed as a consequence.

The strong negative feelings that paedophiles evoke are hard to overcome. You tend to have punitive feelings towards the offender, and the need to maintain a high degree of scepticism can be used to justify an inappropriately aggressive clinical approach. Paedophiles tend to have strong defences of rationalisation and denial. They often feel sorry for themselves and believe that they are the victims. The clinician experiences them as loathsome, self-pitying and self-justifying. Consequently, there is an understandable tendency to keep clinical involvement to a minimum. However, codified medical ethics insist that even paedophiles have a right to appropriate psychiatric treatment. They have to be assessed as objectively as possible. Treatment of a psychiatric disorder occasionally reduces the risk of reoffending.

Mr Jones is a 32-year-old car mechanic. He is under investigation by social services and the police. His seven-year-old stepdaughter has told her grandmother that Mr Jones had intercourse with her when her mother was out. Medical examination has confirmed that intercourse has taken place. Mr Jones does not deny that the child has been abused, but he does deny that he is the abuser. The child has accused him, he claims, because he is stricter than the biological father. She has never accepted him as part of the household. His wife is convinced of his innocence, and as a consequence, the child has been taken by social services and placed in the care of her grandmother. Mr Jones is forbidden to have contact with her, and is not allowed to be alone with any other children. The family is in turmoil, and Mr Jones has approached his GP for psychiatric referral because he has been feeling desperate, and sometimes suicidal, over his situation.

Dr Coltrane has enough information from the referral letter to guess what has been going on. He does not like dealing with this type of situation. He is likely to go into the assessment interview carrying a complex agenda. He wants to avoid colluding with an offender, and therefore he cannot take Mr Jones' account at face value. He is bound to form a judgement as to whether the patient is or is not the abuser. As well as his responsibility to the patient, he has to bear in mind his responsibility to protect other children that Mr Jones may come into contact with.

Within the interview, he aims to be neither obviously hostile, nor uncritically supportive. He has to contain his own feelings of revulsion. He needs firmly to control the interview. If Mr Jones needs treatment, he has to try to establish the basis for a therapeutic relationship. He will have to obtain information from social services before coming to a firm conclusion about the patient. He must consider the possibility that Mr Jones is telling the truth.

There is a further pitfall here. In trying to restrain antagonistic feelings towards a paedophile, it is possible to go too far. The clinician can effectively find himself in a state of denial, whereby he recognises that the patient is guilty of sexual offences against children, but puts this wholly outside of his awareness when dealing with the patient. This can easily lead to a situation in which the psychiatrist colludes with the paedophile, for example by responding to a suicidal crisis by arranging a lengthy inpatient admission that delays a court case for so long that it collapses.

The point of drawing out the problems in assessing people accused of paedophilic offences is that it is obvious that there is no simple solution to the strong feelings they evoke or to the dilemmas in dealing with them. Self-awareness does help, and it can restrain the psychiatrist's most punitive instincts.

Spirituality

We have referred to religion already, but there is a further issue concerning the movement to integrate spirituality into psychiatric care. We must acknowledge that we are major contributors to the controversy over this (e.g. Poole and Cook 2011).

The spirituality and psychiatry movement has significant support amongst mental health professionals in the UK. It has a degree of support from the World Psychiatric Association. There appear to be several different motivations behind the movement:

- There is an assertion that religion and spirituality are important to patients and that psychiatrists have neglected this in the past. Whether or not it has been neglected, it cannot be denied that religion is important to people, and it can be relevant to their mental health problems in a variety of different ways.
- There is a belief that psychiatry has become overly mechanistic and that spirituality brings a more humane and meaningful aspect to mental health care. We disagree that meaning and spirituality are synonymous, but we accept that some clinicians hold the opposing point of view.
- Some techniques based on religious practice may be therapeutically helpful. The key exemplar is mindfulness, which is based upon Buddhist concepts and practices. There is an evidence base for mindfulness and it is certainly helpful sometimes. There is a movement that thinks that many of the ills of Western society can be remedied through mindfulness. This can appear cult-like and it reminds us of the transcendental meditation movement of our youth. We are uncomfortable with it.
- Some argue that having a religious faith is good for your mental health. The evidence for this is highly contentious, and even if it is true, it does not justify the imposition of religious beliefs on patients, which is a serious boundary violation.

This controversy is likely to rage on for some time. Almost everyone agrees that proselytisation is unacceptable in clinical practice. There are unresolved issues over whether it is acceptable to engage in religious practice with patients, such as praying with them. Even psychiatrists who advocate joint prayer urge caution.

The problem with spirituality is that it is not independent of religious belief, and religion often comes with implications about power relationships. In a diverse, multicultural society, psychiatrists need to be aware that aspects of themselves that they experience as benign can have a very different impact on patients. Overt religious affiliation is just one of these.

Main Points in This Chapter

1. All clinicians have values and beliefs that can interfere with therapeutic relationships.
2. Being aware of your own implicit and explicit attitudes is helpful.
3. No matter how strong your beliefs might be, all doctors have to work within the formal ethical code of medicine.

Culture

Culture is a configuration of belief, custom, language, social ritual, values and behaviour, which is held in common by a group of people who identify themselves as distinct from other groups. Culture is the most fundamental of our points of reference in life. It is the filter through which we experience the world. Within our own communities, we are hardly aware of our own culture. Generally speaking, we become conscious of our culture when it is contrasted with a different culture. In other words, we become aware that our cultural assumptions exist only when we meet someone who does not share them.

One of the most attractive features of modern inner cities is their vibrant cultural diversity. Most psychiatrists working in these areas become culturally aware and comfortable with working across cultural divides. The minority of psychiatrists who do not achieve this are of very limited use to their patients. Cultural awareness ultimately teaches you that different peoples have similar underlying needs. Cultural differences can be profound, but people are people. There is much more that unites us than divides us.

Cultural awareness is harder to achieve when working with less diverse populations. It is often those mental health services that have the smallest number of patients from minority ethnic groups that have the greatest difficulty in dealing appropriately with cultural difference. Furthermore, culture is not synonymous with ethnicity. There are significant cultural differences between white middle-class doctors and white working-class patients. It can be hard to be aware of class-based cultural differences.

Transcultural Exotica versus Cultural Awareness

British psychiatry intermittently becomes interested in 'culture bound syndromes'. For example, koro is said to be a manifestation of anxiety that occurs mainly amongst people in South Asia, particularly in Chinese populations. Koro is said to typically affect males. The victim suffers from somatic symptoms of anxiety, and becomes convinced that his penis is retracting into his body, and that this will kill him. Some sufferers try to stop or reverse the retraction process by tying a brick or other heavy object to their penis. There are a number of such culture bound syndromes.

The concept of the culture bound syndrome is not especially helpful. The extent to which such syndromes are bound to a single culture is far from clear. Koro has been reported in a wide variety of populations, including ethnic Europeans, and it can occur in women. There is a worrying implication that it is the bizarre and dramatic quality of koro that makes it interesting. There is an implied Euro-centricity to the effect that Europeans develop core mental disorders only, whilst Africans and Asians develop culture bound syndromes in addition to universal mental illness presentations. There is a post-colonial anthropology here, an implicit suggestion that 'primitive peoples' lack sophistication, and that when they get anxious, they run around with bricks tied to their penises. Not only does this achieve nothing in helping individual patients, it also tends to obscure the true significance of culture, and the subtle ways in which culture shapes mental disorder.

Liverpool has the longest established Chinese community in Europe, and we have worked with this community over many years. Between us, we have only once ever seen one case of koro, and that affected an English teenager with no connection to the Chinese community. However, there are many cultural factors that do influence the presentation and treatment of mental illness in that community. These factors are complex, and generalisations can be misleading. Broadly speaking, there is a Chinese attitude that dictates that you should, as far as possible, avoid contact with authority; that you should cause no trouble and try to be invisible to officialdom. Chinese culture is stoical and uncomplaining. As a consequence, Chinese people tend to be deferential to doctors, and tend to want to be discharged from follow-up as quickly as possible. Chinese people tend not to press an understanding of their culture upon you; you have actively to seek to understand it.

Compared to Europeans, Chinese people have a very different way of understanding emotional and physical well-being. Concepts of balancing opposing influences, of yin and yang, are important. For example, they affect food and diet, which in any case have a particular role in social ritual. Psychotic experiences are often rationalised by Chinese patients as being due to the influence of spirits or ancestors. Whilst beliefs about spirits and ancestors are prevalent in the Chinese community, friends and family have little difficulty in distinguishing psychosis from more ordinary beliefs. Many Chinese people regard mental illness as shameful.

People with mental illness are often intensively cared for by their family, and presentation to services tends to occur very late. People whose disturbed behaviour is loud, difficult and public can find themselves shunned and isolated. The Chinese community in Liverpool does not share a single language, the most common tongues being Cantonese and Hakkar, which are widely spoken in Hong Kong. Mandarin is the official language of mainland China, and since foreign travel has become easier for Chinese people in general, the number of Mandarin speakers in the UK has increased. A significant minority of women have only basic English. Written Chinese pictograms, on the other hand, are not specific to a language, and are universally understood.

It is this type of cultural knowledge, rather than a focus on exotic syndromes, that is worth knowing about, because it facilitates therapeutic relationships with patients from other cultures. It does require that you take the trouble to find out about minority communities.

Urban psychiatrists deal with patients who speak a wide range of languages, and who come from diverse backgrounds. It would be impossible to have prior knowledge of all of these. All psychiatrists have to use translators from time to time, and you have to be prepared to find out about the patient's culture by asking about it directly (Box 10.1).

Working with Translators

The use of translators is essential in many situations where the patient is not fully fluent in spoken English, including where the person has some English. The difference between interpreters and translators is that interpreters bring an element of analysis and explanation to the task. In psychiatry, interpretation is less satisfactory than translation, because the

---

BOX 10.1 Not All Differences Are Cultural in Origin

Dr Holliday is a GP. She is called out at night by a couple to see their five-year-old son. The couple came to the UK from India a year earlier. They are very polite, and obviously relieved to see the doctor. The child is mildly pyrexial, complains of generalised aches and pains, and has a sore throat. He is not unduly distressed, and the only physical finding is inflamed fauces. Dr Holliday is annoyed. The child obviously has a mild viral infection that does not merit a home visit at night. She is tempted to reprimand the family for abusing her availability, but she is curious as to why the parents are so worried. She asks them what they had thought was wrong with the child. They reply that they feared he had rheumatic fever. Rheumatic fever is common in India and it is a major cause of morbidity. Sore throat, joint pains and pyrexia are the presenting symptoms. Their anxiety is reasonable and understandable.

BOX 10.2 A Translation Problem

Mrs Khan is a 55-year-old Pakistani lady. She is referred by her GP to be seen at home by Dr Coltrane. She has taken to her bed over the past two months and she will not get up. She is reluctant to eat and her doctor thinks that she is depressed. Mrs Khan lives with her husband and their extended family in a Victorian terraced house. She speaks no English.

Dr Coltrane is greeted by Mrs Khan's eldest son, who was born in the UK. He explains that his father, who also speaks little English, would like to have a few words before his wife is seen. The elder Mr Khan, using his son as translator, explains that his wife is complaining of weakness, and that she is suffering from a headache. He is worried because it is unusual for her to be ill.

Dr Coltrane goes to the bedroom, which is rather bare. Mrs Khan is huddled under the bedclothes, and she is moaning quietly. Using the younger Mr Khan as translator again, he tries to interview Mrs Khan. Her answers are brief. After 20 minutes, he is not getting very far. He begins to wonder why she is so reluctant to tell him anything, and asks 'Is anyone frightening you?' Mrs Khan is momentarily more animated, speaking and gesturing at some length. Her son translates: 'No'. It is obvious to Dr Coltrane that whatever Mrs Khan said, it was more complicated than 'No'. He presses her son to tell him exactly what she said. He replies that she had said no, and that the rest of the answer was rubbish. Further pressed, he looks embarrassed and laughs uncomfortably. He reveals that Mrs Khan had complained that there are Germans on the roof who talk about her constantly and prevent her from sleeping. Her son takes pains to point out that this is patently untrue. Insisting that all further translation should be verbatim, Dr Coltrane slowly elicits a range of psychotic phenomena.

---

interpreter unwittingly usurps the psychiatrist's role by trying to make sense of things. However, translation is also problematic (Box 10.2). Even the best translators have difficulty in conveying the subtleties and nuances of what is being said. Professional translators are generally better than family or friends. Professional translators are taught to avoid interpreting too much, to avoid organising and thus altering what is said. Family and friends make poor translators. Inevitably, they have their own agenda, and confidentiality is impossible. However, professional translators may come from the patient's own community, and thus may be directly or indirectly known to the patient. This can create real problems. Telephone translation services can get round this, but they are slow and cumbersome to use.

When interviewing someone who identifies themselves as a member of the deaf community, a sign language translator is essential. It is important to know that there is a distinctive deaf culture, although not all people with hearing impairment are part of it (see the discussion of subcultural differences below). It is also important to know that British Sign Language is different to both American and Irish Sign Language, which are similar to each other.

There are some broad principles which are helpful when working with translators:

1. It is better to postpone an interview than to go ahead with an inadequate or inappropriate translator. Delay is usually less of a problem than getting things wrong.
2. Translators need to be told to translate exactly what has been said in each direction. Where this is difficult, they should ask the speaker to rephrase what they have said.
3. Before the interview commences, make sure that the patient is comfortable with the translator.
4. As far as possible, avoid using family and friends as translators.
5. Do not interview the translator. Look at the patient as you normally would in any other interview.
6. Try to keep sentences short, and avoid jargon and colloquial forms of expression.
7. In the course of any translation, some responses to questions will be muddled. It is important to clarify these, to be clear whether the muddle is linguistic or a reflection of the patient's mental state.
8. When conveying information to the patient, say it at least twice in different ways, and ask for it to be repeated back.
9. At the end of interviews, it is worth asking translators for their impression, as at that stage they can safely interpret what has been said, and explain cultural nuances.

Subcultural Difference Related to Class

Communities are not geographical entities. They are groups of people who interact sufficiently frequently to develop a sense of cohesion. In both towns and the countryside, communities exist alongside each other, sometimes with little contact or mutual awareness. In the UK, class is a particularly strong subculture, around which communities form. However, lifestyle can carry the same function. Gay subcultures and communities exist, although not all gay people live within them. Many homeless people live in city centres close to the hub of society's financial and political institutions, with a lifestyle and subculture that is utterly alien to the mainstream of British society.

Homelessness has a very strong association with mental disorder, be it mental illness, substance dependency or personality disorder. It is hard to know whether a significant proportion of single homeless people ever were stereotypical tramps, but they certainly are not now. The middle-aged street drinker, dishevelled and shouting, may live on the streets and use homeless facilities, but they often have accommodation. They gravitate to street drinking because they are not tolerated in pubs or bars. Homeless people tend to be young and white, though this is slowly changing. The only minority ethnic group with major representation amongst the homeless is the Irish. Young homeless people tend to have a background history of family disturbance, and of growing up in the care of adults who were not their biological parents. Some become homeless when they leave the armed forces. Very few live permanently on the streets. They tend to have unstable accommodation, moving between hostels, bed-and-breakfast establishments, bondies (empty buildings), prison and the streets. Most have problems that lead to anti-social behaviour, and exclusion because of this behaviour drives the instability in their living circumstances.

Drug and alcohol misuse is often a major activity, and funding this necessitates criminality and sex work. Exploitation and manipulation of the settled population is an accepted social norm. Although homeless environments are violent and dangerous, homeless people maintain high levels of cooperation, and tend to look after each other. Their decision-making may appear short-sighted, but looking after immediate needs can seem more important than worrying about long-term concerns when you are living under extreme conditions. The degree of mutual support and comradeship in homelessness can make it very difficult to settle in more isolated permanent accommodation, and some people repeatedly choose to return to the streets. It can be hard for middle-class professionals to understand that, despite the deprivation and squalor of homelessness, the lifestyle has some advantages for some people.

Racism

One of the difficulties about being a migrant, a refugee or a member of a minority ethnic group in the UK is that there is a significant chance of being the victim of xenophobia or racism. This does not affect all ethnic minorities and individuals to the same extent. However, it is undeniable that racism is a tangible reality in the everyday lives of a significant proportion of the population living in the UK.

Racism is a complex phenomenon. Some elements are ideological and explicit. They involve direct threats to people's well-being, such as racial harassment and racially motivated violence. Other elements are implicit and unspoken, and they may be invisible to white British people. Examples include the experience of young black men at the hands of the police and the criminal justice system, barriers to employment, and difficulties in securing appropriate housing. Racial tensions exist between different minority ethnic groups, and this too may be outside of the awareness of the majority community.

Racism can be an important part of the context in which black people become mentally ill, and the problems it causes have to be understood. It is highly likely that the experience of growing up with racism accounts for the high rate of psychosis amongst black people born in the UK. Psychiatrists need to be prepared to acknowledge that racism is a tangible reality. There is little point in helping someone to recover from a mental illness as an inpatient, if they are to return to a housing situation where they are constantly racially harassed, as they are unlikely to remain well under such circumstances.

Black patients sometimes accuse individual psychiatrists of being racist. Few psychiatrists regard themselves as racist, and most identify themselves as anti-racists. The accusation may seem tiresome, groundless and offensive. It is hard to form a positive relationship with someone who assumes that you are prejudiced against them from the start. The accusation most commonly arises in the context of a psychiatrist detaining a patient against their will, or making some other unwelcome decision. To the psychiatrist, his or her actions have nothing to do with ethnicity or racism. However, it is understandable that, if you experience racism in your daily life, you are likely to interpret seemingly incomprehensible and unwelcome professional behaviour in the same terms. Understanding this makes it easier to build a therapeutic relationship later.

Just to complicate things, there is racism within mental health services. Our organisations do not stand separate from the rest of society, and there is no reason to expect that health services will be any more or less racist than any other British institution. Some individual members of staff hold racist beliefs, though they are only openly expressed in unguarded moments. Antagonism towards East European migrants tends to be more explicit. Some mental health staff have a very low threshold for believing that people from these backgrounds are feigning symptoms of mental illness. This seems to be related to a dominant view amongst politicians and the media that migrants are often in the UK to secure something to which they are not entitled. The feigned symptom hypothesis is commonly expressed but rarely confirmed amongst any group of patients, and it is a particularly improbable behavioural strategy amongst people who are living in a foreign country and routinely coping with xenophobic hostility. A bona fide mental illness is a much more plausible development.

There are many ethnic minority staff working within the mental health services, but they are disproportionately concentrated in low status jobs. In trying to get past the patient's perception that they may be a racist, the psychiatrist is at a disadvantage if there is obvious evidence of racism in his or her working environment.

BOX 10.3 Not All Problems Have a Satisfactory Solution

Dr Omatayo is a Nigerian psychiatrist who has been working in a UK university department for a year. He is an experienced doctor with a postgraduate qualification in psychiatry. He is working abroad to complete his training, but he is employed as an SHO, which is a post of lower status than the one that he occupied at home. On his first evening on call in an emergency department, a 24-year-old white man is brought in by the police, having been found walking along the central reservation of a dual carriageway. He is agitated and shouting, and he has hit a policeman on the way to hospital.

When Dr Omatayo enters the room, the man spits at him. He then breaks into a rapid and unbroken tirade that is extremely offensive. Neither the police nor the doctor can interrupt or make him listen to any questions. The man makes many racist references to Dr Omatayo, and he complains that Dr Omatayo has been having sex with white nurses outside the consulting room door. He condemns the police for interfering with English people when they should be sending blacks back to their own country. He says that if the police leave, the doctor will castrate him, and he demands to see a solicitor about being forced to see a black doctor.

Dr Omatayo is very shaken by what the man is saying, and by his inability to control the interview. The policemen ask him to leave because, they say, his presence is making the man more aggressive and they fear that he will become assaultive.

Dr Omatayo is now in a dilemma. He has no previous experience of this type of open racism. He is uncertain whether the man is expressing unpleasant but genuinely held views (that is, he does not know if the man is an ideological racist) or whether he is simply very psychotic. The nursing staff are outraged and feel he should not have to put up with this abuse. They suggest that the police should be allowed to take the patient to the police station in order to charge him for the previous assault. The consultant on-call is Indian and it seems likely that he will experience a similar reaction if he tries to interview the man. There appears to be no satisfactory solution.

This is not to say that all black patients approach services with an agenda dominated by suspicion and an expectation of racism. We are not recommending that psychiatrists treat people from ethnic minorities any differently from the rest of the population. Indeed, most people are very happy to be treated the same as everyone else, and only get upset when they feel that this is not the case. The point is to accept and to understand that issues of racism are important. They are distinct from issues of culture.

Special Minorities

There have been continuous attempts to deter displaced people from coming to the UK over the past 20 years. Until recently this was framed as a problem with 'asylum seekers', a term that was coined as an alternative to 'refugee', which might evoke general sympathy. It was tied to the concept that a large proportion of refugees had no genuine fear of persecution and attempted to enter the UK to find work or to claim benefits. The narrative has now changed. At the time of writing, there is a full-blown refugee crisis affecting the whole of Europe and beyond. The terminology has changed in the face of the indisputable evidence that parts of the Middle East are engulfed in an appallingly brutal conflict. It is now argued that refugees should be given little comfort here, as to do so would encourage people to make the dangerous passage across the Mediterranean Sea.

Whether or not you are sympathetic to 'asylum seekers' and refugees, there can be little doubt about the consequences of government policy towards them. They are given very little cash. They are compelled to live in particular places, often 'dispersal centres' in provincial cities. They are prevented from settling into national groupings, and they are frequently very isolated. They can be moved at short notice. Like East European migrants, they are vilified in the press and they are harassed by local people. If they are refused asylum or refugee status, they have no means to support themselves. They may be expected to return to their country of origin, sometimes forcibly. A significant number have experienced torture and other trauma. Some of them develop acute mental illness. It is hard to overcome the combined effects of displacement, loss, impoverishment, communication problems, vilification, traumatisation and insecurity. Working with refugees and asylum seekers creates significant practical, clinical and ethical problems.

There is a parallel with the situation of travellers or 'gypsies'. Although travellers were subject to genocide in the twentieth century, open prejudice against them remains socially acceptable in a significant part of British society. Rural pubs sometimes have signs at the door saying 'No travellers'. Although not necessarily poverty stricken, travellers live quite separate lives, sometimes marked by frequent changes of location. Travellers experience real difficulties in accessing services such as education and health care.

They are often perceived as intrinsically criminal, and they can be subject to severe harassment. Offering even basic mental health services to refugees, 'asylum seekers' and travellers is difficult. It demands that mental health professionals make special efforts to understand the lives, culture and problems of people who are marginalised and vilified. They rarely receive treatment of the same quality as that offered to the rest of the population. In the face of our frank inability to offer a solution to this, we suggest that an awareness of these problems is important.

Main Points in This Chapter

1. Notwithstanding cultural differences, nearly everyone in the world wants and needs the same things.
2. The effects of cultural difference can create problems for the psychiatrist, but they are not impossible to overcome.
3. Xenophobia and racism are realities that cannot be ignored.
4. Not all problems have solutions (Box 10.3). The effects of cultural difference, xenophobia, racism and social marginalisation can make it impossible to offer people an equivalent service to that offered to the rest of the population, but the effort is worthwhile.

Who Should I Be?

Your clinical persona can only draw upon your personality. You cannot successfully develop a wholly contrived psychiatric persona, because the outcome is bound to be affected and uncomfortable. Indeed, the quality of *authenticity* is invaluable, and it is more important than any other individual personal characteristic. It is natural that patients find it easier to trust psychiatrists who seem relaxed, genuine and engaging. There are some other personal qualities that are desirable. These qualities are evident in naturally talented mental health professionals from the day they start training. The rest of us have to cultivate these qualities, which is perfectly possible, as long as you know what they are.

Psychological Mindedness

Psychological mindedness has a particular meaning in psychotherapy, but it also has a more general meaning. It has little to do with the science of psychology. It concerns an ability to think about behaviour in terms of people's emotional lives. It is the ability to empathically understand how people feel, to understand 'what makes them tick'. People who are psychologically minded are good at predicting how other people will behave. They can imagine what it is like to be someone else, and how emotions they have never experienced can affect behaviour. In many ways, psychological mindedness is the opposite of narcissism, where other people are not understood as being fully autonomous, but are experienced as servants of the narcissist's needs.

People who are psychologically minded observe people all the time, not just at work. They notice patterns of interaction and make connections between emotional themes. When they cannot understand other people's behaviour, they generate a range of theories to explain it.

Curiosity and an Ability To Understand Other Lifestyles

The curiosity about other people that is useful in a psychiatrist goes beyond ordinary social interest. It verges on being psychologically prurient. It is an intense interest in other people's biographies and in the ways in which they experience the world. The process of finding out about other people is closely linked to imagining what it must be like to be them, out of which springs an understanding of their lifestyle. Curiosity about other people's lifestyles and life histories goes hand-in-hand with psychological mindedness. It is this curiosity that provides the information to develop psychological mindedness.

Warmth and a Non-Judgemental Attitude

To be a psychiatrist you have to like people. Not everyone does. Some people prefer animals, or motor cars, or computers. Psychiatrists encounter patients from a very wide range of backgrounds. They may disapprove of, or be shocked by, their patients' lifestyles. However, they are not employed to make their patients into better people. They are employed to help them overcome mental health problems, and this is difficult if the therapeutic relationship is affected by disapproval or emotional coldness. Warmth is important to all therapeutic relationships. This is not to say that psychiatrists should be emotionally gushing, hugging their patients and creating friendships with them. The degree of warmth in the relationship has to be compatible with maintaining boundaries. The psychiatrist has to remain capable of making dispassionate and objective judgements. The use of warmth in the relationship is in fact somewhat contrived, in that it is deliberately cultivated to achieve a specific end.

The term 'non-judgemental' is a little misleading. It means that the use of warmth is tempered by a type of neutrality. To be neutral does not imply being entirely uncritical. It is necessary to find a position that is neither censorious nor collusive. This type of neutrality means, for example, that when a male psychiatrist is treating a woman who is a sex worker, she feels comfortable in talking about her lifestyle and she feels that the psychiatrist thinks no less of her than of any other woman. Nonetheless, it must be possible for the psychiatrist to discuss with the patient, at the right moment, the effect that her work is having on her self-esteem and emotional well-being.

Unflappability

Temperamentally anxious psychiatrists tend to make patients feel worse and spread panic amongst mental health teams. In clinical work, the unexpected happens regularly. One of the real challenges of psychiatry is that, no matter how experienced you are, you continue to face novel situations and have extremely difficult decisions to make. It is important to maintain the appearance of calmness and to rise above your own fears, in order to make well thought through decisions. Unflappability does not imply that you do not get anxious. On the contrary, blasé and complacent psychiatrists are dangerous, but you cannot indulge yourself in regularly appearing panicky.

Tolerance of Uncertainty

Psychiatry is full of uncertainty. You rarely know whether a decision has been a good one until long after it has been made. Plans to contain risk are often compromises and they have flaws. Sometimes it takes months or years to understand a patient properly, and you have to make decisions in the interim, in the face of uncomfortable ambiguities. If a psychiatrist finds it difficult to tolerate uncertainty, this is likely to cause problems to themselves and to their patients. He or she is likely to find the job unpleasantly stressful, or may cause significant problems by trying to introduce certainty where none exists, or, most likely, both. No one is entirely comfortable in the face of uncertainty, but you have to learn to put up with it.

Ability to Maintain Boundaries

Some mental health professionals have a good understanding of where professional boundaries lie, but they break them anyway. This is often a recurrent pattern. It usually has its origins in a personal need, a kind of neurotic craving to fill personal emptiness that overrides professional taboos. Professional boundaries have to be profound principles, rules that are constantly in your awareness. Incipient breaches need to ring alarm bells. Maintenance of boundaries needs to be automatic and effortless. If this does not happen, therapeutic relationships are bound to go wrong.

Streetwise

This term, which probably came into British usage through *Starsky and Hutch* circa 1975, still seems to have some currency. Everyone seems to agree that being streetwise is an invaluable asset to a psychiatrist. No one, however, seems to be able to define quite what it is, or how to develop it. It relates to a particular kind of knowingness, a sensitive awareness of some of the tough realities of life as it is lived. It is the quality that allows some people to read a situation, to know that it is unsafe to walk down a particular street on a particular day, where a less worldly colleague would stroll on obliviously and get mugged. It allows some people to easily spot dissimulation and lying, and to recognise a scam. It is not the same as cynicism. Streetwise psychiatrists have better relationships with patients living on the margins of society, because these patients come to recognise that the psychiatrist understands their world. Unfortunately, being streetwise seems to be innate, not learned.

What Am I Getting Out of This?

Mental illness carries stigma. General social attitudes towards mental illness are still tinged with fear and ignorance. A medical degree opens up many career opportunities, and no one is forced to work as a psychiatrist. We make a choice to work in an arena that other people shun. It seems likely that there is something unusual about psychiatrists that makes us want to work with mental illness. It is as well to understand what this is. This is not to suggest that our motivations are pathological. On the contrary, there are bound to be motivations for all unforced career choices, and they are only likely to cause problems to psychiatrists if we fail to understand them. It is only possible to offer an illustrative, rather than an exhaustive, list of possible motivations. They include the following.

Personal Experience of Mental Illness

A significant proportion of psychiatrists have witnessed mental illness in someone close to them, usually a family member, during their early life. A smaller number have been seriously mentally unwell themselves. Across all areas of medicine, many doctors and other health professionals are drawn to their careers after personal experience of serious illness. For some psychiatrists there is a powerful need to understand mental illness. One can speculate that this might be an attempt to resolve the confusion and fear generated by living with a mentally ill relative. Such motivations can run out of control. For example, heroic and excessive efforts to try to rescue patients from their own behaviour can follow the failure to rescue someone in your personal life. On the other hand, some psychiatrists seem to strip mental illness of its emotional content through an excessively reductionist approach. Mental illness becomes nothing more than a dry formula of neurotransmitter dysfunction or automatic negative cognitions (though neither biological psychiatry nor CBT are intrinsically reductionist or emotionless). If you have experienced mental illness as incoherent and frightening in your personal life, it may be comforting to conceptualise it in a more logical and emotionless way. The penalty may be an impairment of empathy and rapport with patients.

Psychological Voyeurism

Some people with severe mental illness exist at the outer limits of human experience. Psychiatrists regularly encounter situations that are outlandish and bizarre. Working as a psychiatrist is often stressful, but it is rarely boring. The work offers unrivalled opportunities for voyeuristic excitement. Psychiatry opens a window on the most hidden aspects of life, and it would be foolish to deny that this is attractive to a lot of psychiatrists.

Related to voyeurism is a fascination with the intellectual puzzle at the heart of psychiatry. The basic nature of mental illness is a scientific, philosophical and social conundrum, which allows endless debate, controversy and theorising. Each patient's problem is a smaller puzzle. Many psychiatrists enjoy the cerebral challenge of their work.

Voyeurism can boil over, and excitement over the bizarre can obstruct taking action to help the person. Voyeurism can be rationalised into, for example, an interest in psychopathology or rare syndromes. Patients can become 'a really amazing case of . . .'. Psychiatry is for patients, not for psychiatrists, and excessive voyeuristic or cerebral interest can invert this.

Fantasies of Omnipotence

Psychiatrists have extensive legal powers over patients. Their opinions are treated with great respect by important social institutions such as the courts. Very unwell patients often make remarkable recoveries as a consequence of treatment. Despite negative stereotypes and a low status within medicine, psychiatrists do wield enormous social power. There is real potential for narcissistic pleasure, and for the psychiatrist to come to feel that he or she is more than an ordinary human being. A cult of personality can develop around charismatic psychiatrists, and this can allow them to become isolated, idiosyncratic and ultimately deviant. Some less charismatic psychiatrists are alone in their omnipotent fantasies, and their teams come to despise them.

Vicarious Care Receiving

Teenage motherhood has a number of causes. It tends to occur in needy, emotionally deprived young women who find vicarious fulfilment of their emotional needs through looking after a helpless but emotionally responsive infant. An attenuated form of this dynamic is widespread in the 'caring professions'. Looking after other people is not just pleasurable because of their gratitude; it often has an element of vicariously meeting a personal need to be involved in a caring relationship. A psychoanalyst would regard this sort of vicarious care-receiving through care-giving as a type of projective identification. It is hardly surprising that it is common in psychiatry, where the degree of emotional engagement with patients is unusually high.

Pseudo-Altruism

Community psychiatry is a form of social medicine, as are general practice and community paediatrics. Severe mental illness is a disease of poverty in much the same way that tuberculosis is a disease of poverty. Anyone can get it, but by and large poor people do.

Psychiatrists tend to work with a stigmatised and deprived population. A desire to champion and help the underdog, a kind of missionary fervour, attracts some doctors to psychiatry. This is a form of pseudo-altruism, as it serves the doctor's need to do good, which is often linked to strong political or religious convictions. This can turn into a self-righteous campaigning zeal, where the difference between the doctor's interests and the patients' interests becomes blurred, and personal axes are ground in the guise of advocacy.

Displacement of Emotional Distress

In a therapeutic relationship, the focus of attention is the patient, who is the one with the illness. This guards a number of boundaries, but in reality, psychiatrists can get ill too. Patients and professionals do not belong to separate categories of humanity. Health professionals of all types are prone to lose sight of this and to feel that illness only happens to patients; that they are protected because they are professionals. Mental health staff can experience the serious mental distress of others, whilst feeling personally invulnerable. Confronted with distressing circumstances in their personal lives, they adopt an intellectualising, unemotional persona, which can be very maladaptive. Their work allows them to displace emotion away from themselves, but there is a penalty. When they do become depressed or otherwise mentally unwell, they are very reluctant to acknowledge it or accept help.

Main Points in This Chapter

1. There is no ideal clinical persona for a psychiatrist. You can only build on who you actually are.
2. Despite this, there are some broad characteristics which are helpful, and which can be cultivated.
3. All mental health professionals meet some of their personal needs through their work. There is a range of motivations for being a psychiatrist, none of which is intrinsically pathological, but all of which can cause problems if they run out of control.

Complicated Interviews

In modern practice, assessments and interviews are frequently conducted outside of the traditional one-to-one clinic model.

Multidisciplinary assessment, interviews with informants and families, and interviews in patients' homes are essential elements of clinical practice. These ways of working can provide a richer, more accurate, assessment. They can lay the foundations of a more constructive relationship with the patient and they can facilitate the development and implementation of complex care plans.

Some aspects of contemporary clinical practice are intrinsically challenging for the clinician. Fragmentary interviews are part of how we all now work. Psychiatrists are regularly confronted with assessment tasks that are seemingly impossible to complete satisfactorily.

12

Interviewing with Other Team Members

In mental health care, multidisciplinary interviewing has been going on for a long time. The traditional mental hospital weekly ward round was a form of multidisciplinary interview, although it was frequently poorly conducted. A large group of professionals, some of them unknown to the patient, held interviews that were dominated by one professional, the consultant psychiatrist. There were often no introductions, and the purpose of the interview was rarely explained to patients, who had to work it out for themselves. The rules of the interview were obscure, and it was easy to humiliate the patient, who was at a severe disadvantage compared with the professionals. Most patients hated ward rounds. Like everything else, multidisciplinary interviewing can be misused.

Even taking this into account, there are a number of circumstances where joint interviews have significant advantages:

- Different disciplines bring different perspectives and skills to interviews. Joint assessment interviews have a stereoscopic quality that can lead to a greater depth of understanding and better assessment.
- Patients with serious mental illnesses and complex needs are likely to benefit from the involvement of more than one type of professional in their care. It makes little sense to put patients through multiple assessments and reviews if this can be avoided. Where disciplines do interviews together, coordination and consistency of treatment is improved, and decision-making can be truly shared.
- A team member sometimes needs help from a different discipline to resolve a problem in the patient's care. For example, a community nurse might need a psychiatrist's expertise to help resolve a problem with medication side effects. One-off consultations are difficult if the team member who needs advice is not present in the room. It is usually best, and most practical, for these interviews to be carried out by the professionals together.
  It ensures that the problem has been properly dealt with, that the solution is appropriate to the overall situation, and that there have been no misunderstandings.

Although there are major advantages to joint interviewing in terms of the quality of assessment and efficient use of time, the presence of two professionals does have a major impact on the patient. Most patients regard different individuals and professionals within a team in rather different ways. Relationships with nurses tend to be more informal than relationships with doctors. Doctors tend to be experienced as more intimidating than social workers. This means that patients may trust some members of the team more than others.

The presence of a trusted professional can greatly enhance an interview. For example, people with schizophrenia come to know their community mental health nurse extremely well, and often place great trust in them. Psychiatrists, on the other hand, tend to be more remote and formal. No matter how pleasant the psychiatrist may be, being interviewed by him or her can be daunting for the patient. Many patients value the support of their community nurse during the interview. The interview is less affected by the patient's apprehensions. The community nurse is likely to be able to bring problems to light that would otherwise have gone unmentioned. The nurse, the psychiatrist and the patient can hold a three-way discussion about problems and plans.

It can, however, go wrong. The intended threesome can split into two conflicting camps. If a patient does not trust either team member, he or she can feel bullied by the two professionals. If the team members do not have a good relationship, the interview can become a struggle between them. The patient and the nurse together can end up feeling browbeaten by the psychiatrist. Patients can feel inhibited from discussing sensitive subjects when there are two professionals in the room. They can develop worries about confidentiality. There is more to successful joint interviews than simply putting three people in a room together and hoping for the best.

Team Work and Team Culture

Joint interviews are difficult to conduct if the two team members do not know each other well. Consultant psychiatrists work with a team for years, and team-working becomes second nature. Team members get to know one another's idiosyncrasies. Over many joint interviews, a joint style develops organically, by trial and error, on the basis of what works. The longer you are a member of a team, the more you affect team culture, and the more comfortable working within that culture becomes.

The problem for psychiatric trainees is that they change jobs frequently. They are constantly getting to know other team members. Team culture varies enormously between teams within the same organisation. Patterns of authority and status do not always conform to job descriptions. Working practices vary because of individual preferences or differences in patient populations.

The psychiatric trainee may find themselves the least experienced member of the team, and the person least familiar with joint interviewing. Nonetheless, because of professional roles and implicit hierarchies (less rigid than in the past, but still extant), other team members may look to the trainee to lead joint interviews. It is important to learn to adjust to unfamiliar working environments as quickly as possible. This requires observation and modelling. Teams lose sight of the idiosyncrasies in their working practices. They forget that teams work differently to each other. They are not well placed to recognise what a newcomer needs to know. The best way to learn about joint interviewing is to let a more experienced professional take the lead, irrespective of whether this cuts across professional status.

People with well-developed skills always make complicated tasks look easy, and make highly structured activities look casual and ad hoc. This is why experienced clinicians can appear effortlessly to resolve previously intractable problems. To the experienced, the structure of joint interviewing is so self-evident that they are hardly aware that they are following it.

Planning the Interview

The key to successful joint interviewing is planning. Where both team members know each other and the patient well, this may require no more than a few moments of discussion just before the interview. Under other circumstances it may require a good deal more preparation than this. No matter how pressed for time you may be, it is always best to have a pre-interview discussion.

Collation of Information

Case notes, even when well maintained, rarely hold all the relevant information, whether they are paper or electronic. In any case, it is difficult to extract information from records quickly, and to separate the relevant from the trivial. Furthermore, team members often have a far more detailed and sophisticated knowledge of the patient than is recorded in the notes. It is advisable to take some time to go over the information that is held by each of you, and to be clear about the reliability, or otherwise, of the information you have. If nothing else, this will ensure that you are both up to date and working on the same information.

Purpose and Duration of the Interview

It is always a good idea to be clear as to why you are seeing a patient, but it is particularly important that team members should have a shared understanding of the purpose of a joint interview. It may be that the interview is a routine review, and that the role of the psychiatrist is simply to hear that things are going well. If they do not know this at the outset, they may be more easily tempted into changing things. Interviews aimed at resolving medication problems, assessing suicide risk or reconsidering diagnosis require different emphases. The team members should try to agree a basic agenda for the interview, establishing those matters that each of them want covered before it is over. They need to agree upon a maximum duration for the interview.

Roles

Finally, there should be an agreement as to who will take the lead in the interview, and who will keep notes. Sometimes both parties have to keep notes. Doctors in the UK cannot delegate note keeping to non-medical staff and they are expected to keep a record of all clinical interviews.

The Interview

At the start of the interview, you should ensure that the patient knows who the professionals are, and why they are present. This may involve an explanation of an unfamiliar role. It is usually helpful to state the purpose of the interview as agreed between the team members. The patient may have a completely different agenda, in which case you need to know about this, and accommodate to it.

Generally speaking the main focus should be on the agreed lead interviewer, who should periodically invite the other interviewer's observations or comments. The other interviewer may want to ask further questions or to take over, and needs to be given an opportunity to do so. This avoids one interviewer intervening in a dialogue and disrupting it. Patients are sometimes keen to talk to the other interviewer, in which case you should adapt to their preference and be prepared to swap roles.

Experienced joint interviewers sometimes use the technique of dialogue between the two professionals. This can be useful under a range of circumstances, as a means of drawing the patient into the professionals' way of understanding the situation. It is not an easy technique to master. There is a risk of patronising, or alienating, the patient. It is probably best reserved for use where the team members know each other well.

Breaks in joint interviews can be helpful, especially where things are not going well. They allow discussion between the interviewers and, where necessary, can help to refocus the interview. When difficult decisions have to be made, for example as to whether a patient should be detained under legal compulsion, such breaks are essential. They allow interviewers to make sure that they agree, and to make plans on what to do if the patient reacts badly at the conclusion of the interview. Such breaks do not arise in one-to-one interviews. At first it can feel unnatural to suggest a break. In fact patients often welcome a break and a cup of tea or coffee, and where the interview has become tense, a break can defuse the situation.

Debriefing

Generally speaking, there should be a brief discussion between the team members after the interview. This allows impressions to be shared, agreement on how secure any conclusions are, and the identification of remaining gaps in information. It also allows feedback between team members on joint interviewing technique. We are in the habit of dictating a letter or note entry in the presence of the other team member, to be audio-typed later. This ensures that both contribute to the document and there is no ambiguity over conclusions or plans.

Main Points in This Chapter

1. Joint interviewing has significant advantages, but it can also be intimidating for patients.
2. Planning the interview is essential.
3. One person should lead the interview.
4. Breaks for discussion are useful when interviews run into difficulties.
5. Debriefing is essential and joint preparation of a letter or note entry is useful.

Interviewing Families and Other Informants

The ability to conduct successful interviews with patients' families and friends is a fundamental psychiatric skill. Theoretical aspects of family interviewing are drawn mainly from family therapy practice, and they can be dauntingly complex. There are several distinct family therapy traditions (for example, systemic, behavioural and structural), which use different approaches to family interviewing. Psychiatrists need a small repertoire of generic family interviewing skills in order to conduct routine family and informant interviews confidently and effectively. Experience builds skills, and family theory is far more useful to the experienced interviewer than to the beginner. This chapter is concerned with the basics of family interviewing.

The main reasons for routine family interviewing are:

- To gather information about the patient that they are unable to give themselves, and to verify certain types of information.
- To have a dialogue with the family about the nature of the mental illness, about treatment plans and to discuss what they can do to help.
- To assess relationships and overall family functioning.
- To assess the impact of the patient's illness and behaviour on those around them, especially on carers and children.
- To establish and maintain a relationship whereby professionals and family can work together to help the patient.

In most of medicine, doctors have a tendency to regard talking with families as a chore that is a distraction from the main task of treatment. Psychiatry on the other hand has a marked tendency to locate the origins of mental illness within the family. Child abuse, high expressed emotion and genetics are all primarily family phenomena. Irrespective of the contribution that these factors may make in causing or sustaining mental ill health, families and friends are important in patients' lives. Professionals are transient figures, but families are forever. No matter how far a person migrates socially or geographically, no one can escape the internalised influence of their family of origin. It is important that mental health services are able to work positively with families, irrespective of whether we approve of their lifestyle and values or not.

Families and friends are often profoundly affected by the patient's condition, and in any case, they have their own needs. This can make family interviews highly charged and emotional, and there is a real risk of conflict with the clinician. It can be hard to follow the discussion because different family members have different opinions, and because they follow habitual patterns of family interaction, which follow all kinds of unspoken rules and

---

BOX 13.1 Families Are Systems

Families are small social systems. The membership of a family alters only slowly and families tend to follow stable rules of interaction. Family systems face many threats to their stability and integrity. Family members die. Children grow up and adults grow old, which changes the way that they behave. Conflict occurs from time to time, or it may be continuous. Families have to cope with children leaving home. These are internal and intrinsic sources of family instability. There are also external threats, for example disease, unemployment or infidelity.

To prevent family systems disintegrating in response to these threats, they have homeo-static mechanisms that resist change, and adaptive mechanisms that incorporate change when it cannot be resisted. A system cannot maintain a stable configuration without such mechanisms. A family would break up as soon as it faced any serious problem if it did not have them. When threats arise, the family system tries to find an adaptation that involves minimal change. For example, the loss of a parenting role when children marry may be replaced by an attenuated parenting role with grandchildren. Maintaining the stability of a family is a high priority for its members.

During the process of finding a partner, settling down and forming a new family, there are powerful forces that drive people to reproduce patterns of interaction that are familiar from their family of origin. These patterns are comfortable. We tend to choose partners who are like ourselves and who come from similar families. Most people, when dealing with their children, have the disturbing experience of acting and speaking just like their own parents, despite trying to avoid this. New patterns of family behaviour can rarely be created through an act of will.

Interactions within families follow idiosyncratic and unspoken rules. They are often based upon family myths, which include shared beliefs about the family. For example, a family myth might be that the expression of anger is extremely destructive. This might lead to a rule that anger must not be verbalised. An adverse consequence might be that anger is expressed by protracted sullen silence and that conflict resolution is difficult.

Individuals can come to play special roles within families. For example, children who are hard to discipline can become the scapegoat for everything that goes wrong within the family ('Your mother and I are splitting up because of you'). Successful offspring can come to carry the whole family's aspirations for self-improvement. They may then find it difficult to lower their personal ambitions when the need arises.

When it is hard to understand why families are behaving as they are, it can be useful to consider whether these kinds of factors might be shaping their behaviour.

---

assumptions. Protecting boundaries can be difficult, as families may not see why they are important or relevant. Families sometimes come to interviews with an agenda dominated by a desire to influence the professional's assessment of the patient, or a wish to influence decision-making in order to achieve a particular outcome. The family and the clinician can end up taking rhetorical positions that cannot be reconciled (see rhetorical interviews in Chapter 16).

It can sometimes be helpful to think of families as systems, rather than just as groups of individuals. Some ideas that we have found useful are set out in Box 13.1.

Before the Interview

It would be a betrayal of the therapeutic relationship to talk with a third party about a patient without their knowledge. The clinician has to get the patient's permission first, and this should be documented. In family interviews, the distinction between gathering and giving information is not entirely clear-cut. There is a need for clarity as to whether there are matters that the patient does not want disclosed. There are legal and ethical obligations on any doctor in these situations. Conversely, where the patient is happy for information to be given, there is no excuse for withholding it from the family.

There are some complexities with regard to the patient's consent. Firstly, in the UK, under certain circumstances, there is a legal obligation to consult with relatives prior to legally detaining the patient. Secondly, where there is a significant element of risk, or in order to assess someone who is seriously unwell, it may be necessary to override their explicit wishes and take information from informants. Thirdly, where a third party is at risk, it may be necessary to break confidentiality. This is a legal obligation if a child is at risk. There may also be a legal obligation to warn an adult who is a potential victim where there are, for example, jealous delusions. These breaches of professional boundaries should not be taken lightly, and must be capable of justification to the patient, even if they are unlikely to agree that it was warranted. Where breaches of confidentiality occur, the reasons for this should be documented, and the patient should be told about it as soon as is practicably possible.

If you are interviewing more than one person, it is best to have two interviewers in the room. Family interviews are potentially complicated situations, and it is difficult to conduct the interview and observe what is going on at the same time. Naturally enough, the considerations about joint interviewing set out in Chapter 12 apply. It is particularly important for the team members to be clear about their agenda, the length of the meeting and who is going to lead the interview.

In general, patients should be included in family interviews, even where this is awkward. Openness is always the best governing principle, even when it makes things difficult in the short run. Taking the line of least resistance by excluding the patient often leads you to a much more difficult and dishonest position in the long run. Nonetheless the problems of including the patient in the interview are sometimes very real. Patients who are actively unwell, especially those who are manic or suffering from psychosis, can find family interviews stressful. They may become disturbed during the interview as a consequence. Family members can find some matters very difficult to talk about in the presence of the patient, including simply stating that they think they are mentally unwell. Generally speaking, patients should only be excluded if this is their own wish or if there is a real risk of tangible harm occurring if they are included. Certainly, the psychiatrist should never say anything to a family that he or she would not be happy to say in the same way to the patient.

At the Start of the Interview

Following first principles, introductions are important. Families and friends are often unfamiliar with professional roles, and saying 'I'm the CT1' or 'I'm an OT' may convey nothing to them at all. 'I'm the doctor based on the ward' or 'I'm an occupational therapist and I work with people on their daily living skills' is much more meaningful. The family must be told how long the interview will last, but they should always be told that there will be further opportunities to meet. 'One-off' interviewing creates an intolerable pressure on a family to deal with everything that matters to them within that interview.

Introductions need to be made in both directions. It is essential to know who everyone is, and the nature of their relationship with the patient. Sometimes, family members bring their friends to support them; the friend has a relationship with the patient's relative but not with the patient. You need to know this.

At this stage, before the discussion has started, you have to state that there are limitations to what you can disclose. Families have long-standing and deep relationships with patients, and, understandably enough, they rarely see why the rules of confidentiality should apply to them. Patients, on the other hand, often want confidences kept from those closest to them. Acknowledging that something is being withheld creates a partial disclosure. Consequently, confidentiality has to be raised as a principle, rather than waiting until you cannot answer a question (thus revealing where a secret lies).

Having completed these preliminaries, it is important to set out an explicit agenda for the meeting. This involves stating clearly what you hope to achieve in the course of the interview, and inviting the family to do likewise. Where they do not have a clear agenda, and even where they do, it can be useful to ask each of them how they see the patient's problem. The question often exposes misunderstandings, undisclosed items of history and a range of other significant information.

If there seems to be an unrealistically huge joint agenda, the family can be asked to identify the two or three matters that are most important to them. Other agenda items can be dealt with at a later meeting.

During the Interview

Controlling Family Interviews

If you have prepared the ground properly, the majority of routine family interviews are straightforward. They are not generally difficult to control. There is often a family spokesperson, who does most of the talking. From time to time, it is good to invite other family members to say what they think, or to ask whether they agree. This ensures that all views can be aired. It can also help unlock the discussion, should it start going in circles.

All psychiatrists will occasionally have difficult interviews with families, and the experience can be quite aversive. Families sometimes come feeling defensive, aggrieved or guilty. They may be angry with the psychiatrist, with the patient or with each other. It may not be clear exactly who it is that they are angry with, or why. All of these can make it difficult to have a fruitful interview. The presence of a number of angry people in the room can be very uncomfortable. Although it is very uncommon for real aggression to emerge, it is not helpful to continue if emotions are running out of control. It is important to recognise when an interview has become counterproductive and to close it.

There are two techniques that can disarm conflict in family interviews. These are positive connotation and acknowledgement of fallibility.

Positive connotation means that the behaviour of family members is acknowledged by the interviewer as being well-intentioned. This stance is maintained even with regard to behaviour that the psychiatrist feels is misguided or counterproductive. Behaviour is not directly criticised, but is construed as the consequence of family members attempting to do their best under difficult circumstances. This has the advantage of almost always being true. Even when it is not strictly true, it can free defensive family members from feeling attacked. It is intended to place the clinician outside of the family dynamic, as he endorses everyone equally.

Acknowledgement of fallibility is an interpersonal strategy that runs counter to medical culture. It seems self-evident that one should admit mistakes and apologise for them.

Explanations and apologies tend to avoid severe problems in relationships, complaints and litigation. In the NHS, doctors have a formal duty of candour, but this has yet to alter prevailing attitudes and doctors have to work at this.

Acknowledgement of fallibility involves more than simply putting your hands up to genuine errors. It also involves expressing regret over (or apologising for) incidents and factors that are outside of your control. For example, in the face of serious mental illness, families' distress can focus on relative minutiae. Consequently, families may have grievances that seem 'unreasonable'. In a high risk situation leading to compulsory admission, they may complain about the involvement of the police. They may protest that a previously highly aggressive patient now seems rather drugged. It is helpful to acknowledge that such matters are distressing, and sometimes to apologise for them, even though they are an inevitable or appropriate part of the treatment process. This is not to say you can disown these aspects of care. You certainly should never imply that someone else's conscientious actions were inappropriate. The recognition that the treatment is imperfect and that you are fallible is both true and disarming in many circumstances. The ability to strike this position requires professional self-confidence, and is rarely possible if you feel significant defensiveness over what has happened.

Obtaining Information from Families

Family interviews are unusual settings. Answers to questions can be corrected or debated by family members. Compared with individual interviewing, a family interview often provides a clearer and richer picture of how things have developed. A clinical hypothesis can be tested by putting it to the family, and asking them what they think.

In gathering information, it is important to focus on events and specific behaviours. Families will often talk about feelings and causal theories. This is natural enough, but the psychiatrist needs to know what has actually happened and specific examples of behaviour, so that the context and the sequence of events can be fully explored.

Sometimes you want to know about patterns of behaviour within families. This can be useful in assessing, for example, the degree to which the patient is exposed to emotionally arousing responses from family members. It is usually best to ask a third person within the family about the interaction between two other family members. The third person is likely to have a clearer view of the interaction, and is more likely to be able to describe it without re-enacting the emotions. For example, a sibling can be asked about a parent's responses to the patient. The two participants are more likely to tell you how the other makes them feel than what they actually do. In any case, they may not be aware of their own habitual patterns of response. The process of asking one family member about the interactions between two other family members can be repeated with respect to each dyad in turn. This even-handed process can reveal a great deal about the way that a family functions. This is called circular questioning.

Sometimes, it is possible to infer aspects of family functioning from behaviour in the interview. For example, patterns of dependency, hostility or alliance may be revealed in the choice of seating positions, and responses to distress say something about the quality of relationships. Family beliefs, myths and rules may be implied during the interview. However, it is important to bear in mind that these are always inferences, which should normally be tested by asking the family about the accuracy of the observation. Families do not always interact normally in the presence of a psychiatrist.

> **BOX 13.2** 'Don't Tell Her We Told You, but She's Planning to Kill Gran'
>
> Caroline is a 20-year-old student. Her family has noticed that for over a year or so she has become increasingly suspicious and irritable. Eventually, she takes a serious overdose. On assessment, she is found to have symptoms of acute schizophrenia, and she agrees to be admitted to hospital. Several days later, her mother phones the ward doctor, Dr Smith. She is very worried, and wants to tell Dr Smith something in strict confidence. She has been reading her daughter's diary. Caroline has written several entries to the effect that her grandmother has been replaced by a demon and that she must be killed in order to restore her true grandmother. There was a kitchen knife with the diary. The old lady is disabled by heart disease and lives in the household.
>
> Caroline's mother is extremely concerned about the welfare of both her daughter and her own mother. However, she does not want to do anything to jeopardise her relationship with Caroline, as she realises that Caroline is going to need her family's support over the next few years. She does not want their daughter to know that she has been going through her possessions. She does not want Caroline to feel that she thinks she is a potential murderer. If Dr Smith mentions the contents of the diary, Caroline will know that the information could only have come from her mother. She does not want the diary to be directly mentioned. Naively, she believes that the knowledge that the entries exist will allow the psychiatrist to assess and contain her daughter's dangerousness.
>
> Dr Smith is in a difficult position. Caroline's mother has good reasons for secrecy, albeit based on some misconceptions about the abilities of psychiatrists. However, she can only explore the information by confronting Caroline with the contents of the diary, in breach of her undertaking of confidentiality to her mother.

There is a very common problem that arises in family interviews, and that is the conditional disclosure of information. An example is set out in Box 13.2. It can be hard to understand why families want to conceal the fact that they have made a disclosure. The risk of an argument or of unpleasantness often seems trivial in the face of the importance of the information disclosed. However, there are all kinds of barriers to frankness within families, and there is often more at stake than is immediately obvious.

When a family member is mentally unwell, relationships can feel very fragile. Disclosure of secrets carries a higher than usual risk of breakdown of relationships and it therefore threatens the integrity of the family. Disclosures may involve breaking family rules (for example, 'We don't tell outsiders our business'). Families have sometimes colluded with the patient, for example by agreeing with them that delusions are true. Having avoided conflict in this way, a disclosure risks revealing that the collusion was dishonest and that effectively they have been lying to the patient for weeks or months.

Although families request undertakings of confidentiality for reasons that are salient, wherever possible you should decline to make an undertaking to conceal a disclosure prior to it being made. There are two good reasons for this. Firstly, families often suppose that once the psychiatrist knows the information, he or she has some power to get the patient to talk about it. In fact, it is almost always impossible to do anything with the information unless you can confront the patient with it. Secondly, concealment introduces dishonesty between the psychiatrist and the patient, and this can cause problems later, for example when the information appears in a report.

If these reasons are explained most families will understand, and they will withdraw the demand for confidentiality about the disclosure. Dealing with the problems caused by disclosure becomes a joint task for family and professionals. However, some families remain very perturbed. Occasionally, as there is no strict duty of confidentiality to the family, you have to go ahead and tell the patient anyway. Even if it is possible to observe the family's wishes without adverse consequences, you can never make an unconditional undertaking to withhold information from a patient. There is always a possibility that circumstances will arise where you have to tell.

Giving Information to Families

In giving information to families, it is particularly easy to make an assumption about what they already know and hence accidentally break confidentiality. You cannot assume that all family members know what you know, and even apparently innocuous information can be very sensitive in some families. You should only give information when you are clear about the family members' understanding of the situation, knowing what information is common currency and what is not. It is important to go slowly, with lots of repetition.

At the End of the Interview

At the end of the interview, there is an opportunity to give any message that you particularly want the family to hear, which will usually be a reiteration of something you have said earlier. You should not underestimate how easily messages can be misinterpreted in these interviews, no matter how intelligent the participants may be. Consequently, important messages need to be stated very clearly and simply. It can be helpful to invite the family to make any closing observations or remarks; families will often come up with novel solutions to problems if given the opportunity. Generally speaking, it is helpful to invite the family to meet with you again if they want to, and to state that they may forget what you have said and that you do not mind going over it again at a later date.

Finally, team members need to debrief and reflect on the interview, in order to share observations and to make a record of the interview. If a new hypothesis about the patient or the family emerges, this needs to be recorded, together with a record of the evidence supporting it. The record should state clearly what information the family have been given and any undertakings that have been made to them, for example with respect to future meetings or to avoid certain treatments. When relationships with families go wrong, it is invaluable to have a contemporaneous record of what was said to them. It can help to rescue the relationship.

Accompanied Patients

Patients sometimes arrive at interviews unexpectedly accompanied by a family member or friend. This is usually an attempt to support an anxious patient, although sometimes the family member wants to influence the interview. Occasionally, the family member is an unwelcome and intrusive presence. The interviewer must try to have some time alone with the patient, either at the beginning or end of the interview. Without this, it is impossible to know how the patient feels about the relative's presence, and there is a risk that the interview will be very misleading.

It is reasonable to ask to see the patient alone to begin with. A clear statement at the beginning that the relative will be invited in later will usually avoid attempts to force a joint interview. Very anxious patients may resist this, and the relative may have been invited exactly to avoid seeing you alone. In this case there is no option but to see the pair together. Towards the end, when the patient has relaxed, they may be willing to be seen without the relative for the final part of the interview. What you must avoid is the situation where the patient is never seen alone over several interviews. In our experience, this nearly always leads to the relative's agenda overwhelming and submerging one or all of the patient's concerns.

Children and Carers

Mental illnesses do not just happen in people's minds, they happen in their lives. Severe mental illnesses have a major impact on families. It is well recognised that those who care for people who are mentally ill, usually family members, experience high levels of stress and are vulnerable to becoming depressed themselves. They can become very isolated. They need information, support and a life of their own. When carers do become depressed, this can have an adverse impact upon the patient's mental health, setting up a vicious circle of stress and mental illness.

It is important that mental health professionals should be attentive to carers' needs. Families mostly provide care without question and they tend not to express their needs. Mental health professionals have to have a high awareness that carers may be struggling. The patient's interests and the carer's interests can be in conflict. When a carer is offered an assessment of their own needs, this should be dealt with by a different team (or where this is impossible, a different team member), and independently of the assessment of the patient's needs. Since the Carers Recognition and Services Act 1995, carers in the UK have a right to an independent assessment of their needs, and their rights have been strengthened by several subsequent Acts of Parliament.

Not all families are benign or well-intentioned. They may, for example, exploit the patient in a variety of ways. Malignant families create real dilemmas for clinical teams, as it can be hard to curtail their activities and impractical to get them out of the patient's life. When it is impossible to work with a family, it is nearly always necessary to involve social workers and to use legislation designed to protect vulnerable adults.

Child protection procedures exist to prevent children from coming to serious harm. In the UK, and in much of the rest of the world, there is a legal obligation to place the needs of children over the needs of adults. Child protection is a formal and overriding responsibility of all health professionals, even where the child at risk is unknown to the professional, or where the risk is to children in general. There are no ethical or legal exceptions.

You are obliged to have a low threshold for initiating formal assessment of a patient's child. This can mean serious disruption to the therapeutic relationship with the patient, but it cannot be avoided. If you have a high threshold for referral, then some children will suffer avoidable harm. This is not to say that mentally ill parents necessarily represent a risk to their children or are poor parents, as this is far from the truth. In the course of a career, however, all psychiatrists will come across some patients who are both.

The impact of parental mental illness on children is more far-reaching than the kind of problems that require action under child protection procedures. When the patient has dependent children, the effects of mental illness and of psychiatric treatments are amplified.

Mentally ill parents sometimes do things that frighten their children. Suicide attempts leave children feeling insecure. Sedative side effects of medication and preoccupation with psychiatric symptoms make it difficult to function as a parent, and children lose important parental attention. Often, the other parent is distracted and unavailable to the children. These problems can be quite protracted, and they occur whilst the child's development presses on regardless. Consequently, the effects can be persistent.

Western culture has a strong tendency to try to protect children from unhappiness through denial. For example, children are frequently excluded from unhappy family events, such as funerals. In a similar spirit, families pretend to children that mental illness and hospitalisation are not happening, or that they are insignificant. The adults are often frightened by mental illness, and do not understand it. This makes it difficult to offer the children an explanation, and it is easier to avoid the subject. In fact, even young children are usually aware of parental mental illness.

Community mental health teams (CMHTs) have to attend closely to the needs of their patients' children, and have a role in ensuring that practical steps are taken to avoid emotional harm. This is far below the threshold that triggers child protection procedures. Low-key interventions are far from 100 per cent protective, but they achieve more than doing nothing at all. Above all, children need help to understand what has happened. They do not necessarily need specialist intervention. Children can and should be included in family interviews. Someone in the team has to take the trouble to explain to the family how they can tell the children what has happened in terms that they can understand. If the family cannot do this, a team member may have to do it for them. Once it is recognised that the children's needs should be attended to, the interventions are relatively simple.

Adolescent Patients and Their Families

General adult psychiatry has its origin in large mental hospitals. Child psychiatry has its origin in the child guidance movement of the first half of the twentieth century, which was based on social work and psychotherapeutic practice, both of which were influenced by psychoanalysis. This is one of a number of reasons why general adult and child psychiatry practice are very different to each other.

The twenty-first century has seen the development of adolescent psychiatry services that straddle the conventional age boundaries of childhood and adulthood, together with Early Intervention services that aim to treat psychosis in the prodromal or first-episode stages. Early Intervention and adolescent services are usually targeted at the same age group, roughly 14–24 years.

These developments blurred the boundaries between previous age-determined services, which is a good thing. The involvement of families in the care of adolescent patients can be tricky. Adolescent services tend to emphasise the autonomy of their patient, which can mean excluding families from involvement. However, this cuts the team off from direct knowledge of the environment that is most important to the patient. Understanding a patient's early developmental history without talking with their parents is difficult, as there is invariably salient information from the early years that the patient does not know.

There are real dilemmas here, but in our experience it is very difficult to work successfully with young people who are developing a psychotic illness without the involvement of their family. Autonomy is a sensitive issue for adolescents, so that pressing for contact with the family has to be done tactfully, but the alternative of working solely with the patient is akin to driving a motor vehicle when blindfolded. A successful outcome is possible, but it is mainly due to luck.

Long-Term Relationships with Families

Just as therapeutic relationships can last for a long time, so too can relationships with patients' families. The vast majority of these relationships are helpful and of good quality. Occasionally, the relationship with the family is better than the relationship with the patient. The professionals and the family start routinely to conspire to manipulate the patient. Tempting though this can be, it is a betrayal of the relationship with the patient, which then can never be improved, even if a new team takes over.

Occasionally, families turn out to have attitudes towards the patient or his illness that are overindulgent, neglectful or bizarre. It is very tempting to avoid confronting these attitudes in the interests of sustaining the relationship with them. This is usually a mistake. If you do not tackle such problems at the beginning of the relationship with the family, it is generally impossible to do anything about it later. Challenging family members need not be aggressive, but there should be a clear statement of disagreement. For example, if parents believe that individual psychoanalysis is the treatment of choice for their daughter's schizophrenia, going along with the idea on the basis that there is a long waiting list for psychotherapy will tend to create a difficulty when the daughter eventually comes to the top of it. An early statement of disagreement may be awkward, but it serves the patient's interests much better in the long run.

Finally, you have to bear in mind that families are systems that can only be imperfectly understood. When a professional gives information to a family, it can have an unexpected impact. It may alter perceptions as to the nature and causes of the patient's problems. This can, in turn, significantly alter interactions within the family. Altered interactions can be helpful, but they can also destabilise families. Marriages that have survived years of difficult behaviour may abruptly break down if a psychiatrist changes the family's view of the patient's responsibility for their own actions. There is little that you can do to prevent this, but you have to anticipate that unexpected responses to family interviews will sometimes happen.

Main Points in This Chapter

1. Families, even dysfunctional ones, are important to patients, and you have to be able to work with them.
2. Families are systems with homeostatic mechanisms. This may explain some aspects of family behaviour.
3. Family interviews require the patient's consent. The patient should participate.
4. It is easy accidentally to breach confidentiality in family interviews.
5. A handful of special techniques, such as circular questioning, positive connotation and acknowledgement of fallibility, make difficult interviews a lot easier.
6. Disclosure of information should not be accepted on a conditional basis.
7. Patients' families, especially their dependent children, have important needs. A small amount of attention to these can make a big difference.
8. Recovery from mental illness is more likely where there is a three-way alliance between family, patient and professionals.

In the Community

Why Bother To Interview Patients at Home?

Psychiatry developed within large institutions, and the clinical practice of psychiatry still bears a clear imprint of its institutional origins. British mental hospitals have closed or are greatly shrunken, and whilst repeated efforts have been made to eliminate the patterns of working that developed there, they endure in many of the new, smaller, more dispersed facilities. A small proportion of older members of the profession are nostalgic for the certainties of a working life in the asylums. There are pressure groups that campaign for a return to more institutional, and custodial, forms of care.

This attachment to the past seems to us to be extraordinary, as the evidence for the superiority of community psychiatry over institutional psychiatry is overwhelming. Institutional psychiatry was disliked by patients and caused secondary limitations to functioning. Asylum staff were well-intentioned, and the asylums were the best form of care available at the time. However, the institutions became barren places to live, and many chronically unwell patients experienced empty and wasted lives, their symptoms worsened by the environment that was supposed to be helping them to recover.

The perception that community psychiatry is associated with an increased risk to patients and the public has little basis in empirical evidence. In our opinion, the perception has probably arisen because, with the closure of asylums, adverse incidents that once passed unnoticed behind institutional walls now occur in public view. Our attachment to community psychiatry may be in part based on our personal dislike of hospitals, but it has strong support from the evidence base and from humanitarian considerations.

In the twenty-first century, British psychiatry is in an odd state of development. After a lengthy period of investment in community services, economic austerity has brought service reductions. In England, marketisation of the NHS has uncoupled previously well-integrated health and social care. There are multiple models of care across the UK and it is hard to generalise about them. It would be fair to say that we have physically left the asylums and we are in the community but it is far from clear that everyone is practising what could reasonably be described as fully developed community psychiatry.

The core issue is this: in order to practise community psychiatry, the psychiatrist has to leave the office. This cannot be done by proxy. The fact that the psychiatrist works with other staff who visit the patient at home is insufficient to secure the advantages of community practice. The whole team has to work within the community it serves. Community psychiatry involves assessing and treating patients in their own environments, primarily within their own homes. This brings changes in perspective and an alteration in power relationships. Taking the psychiatrist to the patient rather than vice versa changes everything.

The underlying process of conducting an interview with a patient at home is not significantly different from an office-based interview. It does require a good understanding of multidisciplinary and family interviewing, but the actual skills deployed are unchanged by location. However, within the patient's home there is a very different type of information available regarding their habits, tastes, routines, lifestyle and social environment. Every home environment is individually created (though not necessarily by one person), and they come to reflect profound personal characteristics. No matter how long you talk to a patient and informants in an office, a mass of qualitative information is lost, which can only be accessed by actually going to their home.

In order to utilise this rich source of information, it has to be noticed. Some people notice things more easily than others, but it is also a skill that can be developed. Noticing involves an active curiosity, and has to be linked to a willingness to ask 'why?' Noticing includes, for example, both understanding that personal collections of books reveal important patterns of interests and that a construction of an empty plastic bottle, silver foil and drinking straws is a bong (or crack pipe). There is information evident in a patient's home that can save time by providing answers to standard history taking questions. There are new and different types of information available: powerful, accurate and enduring snapshots of the patient's life.

The other big advantage of community interviewing is that there is a major, though complicated, difference in the relationship between the psychiatrist and the patient from the outset. Psychiatrists sometimes have to exert control over patients, and they routinely try to persuade them to do things that they do not want to do. However, the overarching long-term task is to get alongside the patient, to work together towards the restoration of independence and autonomy. Control is most easily achieved in the psychiatrist's environment, but control is a short-term objective. Getting alongside patients is more easily achieved in the patient's environment.

There is nothing particularly strange or surprising about this. To take a simple example, psychiatrists often run late. There is a significant difference between the patient being kept waiting for half an hour in an unfamiliar waiting room full of strangers, and being kept waiting for half an hour in their own home. The former is stressful and aversive. The latter is, at worst, a minor inconvenience.

Inviting someone into your home means that the interview is proceeding on your territory and, psychologically, on your terms. Many patients who would never agree actively to go to see a psychiatrist in their office will allow you to visit them at home. There is a major difference between agreeing to a psychiatrist visiting to see if they can help, and making the more positive decision that you need to see a psychiatrist and then taking the trouble to go and see them. People usually come to your house to offer you a service. In contrast, a visit to a hospital or to a doctor's surgery places the patient in a more subservient and supplicant position.

So, the simple change of location changes the relationship, such that it is easier to form a cooperative partnership with the patient as opposed to a relationship where the psychiatrist tries to get the patient to bend to his or her will. One reason for trying to get alongside patients, rather than dominating them, is that it works better. People, generally speaking, do not like being told what to do. They are much more likely to follow an agreed plan that they have helped to formulate with the psychiatrist.

Better information and a different type of relationship come with community interviewing, and it allows a team to deal with emergencies differently and to avoid inpatient admissions. It is far easier to treat someone who is psychotic at home if you have seen their home and met their family and friends. Risk assessment is more accurate, and plans can be agreed and implemented immediately. Inpatient admission is the part of psychiatric treatment which is most disliked by patients, and it is far easier to avoid it if the psychiatrist and the rest of the team see the patient at home.

Some types of psychiatric problem can only be properly assessed in the patient's home. For example, the day-to-day functioning of patients with dementia is not necessarily closely correlated with the objective cognitive deficit. It is their ability to cope in their home that forms the most important part of the assessment. There can be a significant difference between the patient's general orientation and their orientation in their home environment. Routine tasks, such as preparation of food, can be witnessed and critical safety issues, such as the patient's ability to operate gas appliances, can be tested. A clinic assessment might accurately reveal the degree of objective cognitive impairment, but it is very difficult to accurately assess functional ability in that setting. People with cognitive impairment tend to function at their worst in hospitals, which is why old-age psychiatrists were the pioneers of home assessment.

There are many further advantages to working in the community, but it must be acknowledged that there are also some significant problems.

Confidentiality

Confidentiality faces novel threats when you work in the community, and it is easy to get caught out. For example, it is easiest to arrange a visit through a telephone call, which is no problem if the patient lives alone. However, if you call and a different family member answers, you may immediately breach confidentiality by giving an honest response to the reasonable question 'Who is calling?' Some traps can be avoided (for example, by writing to the patient and inviting them to call you to arrange an appointment), but some cannot. For example, because of the strong relationship between deprivation and serious mental disorder, in any community psychiatrist's patch, there is likely to be a concentration of patients in certain locations. After a short while in the job, all anonymity is lost, and you are quite likely to be spotted and identified whilst waiting at a doorstep. Even if you are not personally identified, within an inner city community an unknown man in a suit is likely to be spotted and taken to be a police officer or a bailiff. There are likely to be questions about your identity.

Intrusiveness

Most patients prefer to be seen at home, but a few prefer office interviews. One reason is exactly the type of breach of confidentiality set out above. A variety of other factors, such as previous experience of involuntary admission, shame over neglected accommodation or the presence of domineering relatives, can mean that the patient finds the prospect of a home visit intrusive. For this reason, patients have to have the option of an office visit if that is their preference; though under these circumstances it is always important to try to understand what is driving their reluctance to be seen at home. It is likely that the reasons will be important in understanding the patient, and it is often possible to reassure them sufficiently to allow a later home visit.

Lack of Control of the Environment

The main problem with lack of control over the environment is that full control of the interview is more difficult. Other family members may unexpectedly be present, and it can be difficult to get them out of the room (it is their home, after all). Even if they agree to leave the room, they may be able to overhear the interview, which can be inhibiting for the patient and the interviewer alike. It can mean that an assessment is only partially completed. Although there is usually an opportunity to complete the process at a later time, it complicates basic information gathering. There is no doubt that it is better to get the task completed in a single session, not least because the patient is likely to be anxious to hear your opinion. However, in the community, assessment often has to be carried out in phases. This requires clarity about what you have omitted and what you do not know, both of which should be clearly recorded in the notes.

Under many circumstances, the unexpected presence of other family members can be opportunistically exploited, for example in order to get an informant history. It is generally better to utilise the opportunities present in the situation as you find it, rather than ploughing on with your original agenda under circumstances that make it difficult to achieve. Conversely, the presence of small children is much less problematic in the patient's own home than in a clinic setting, as they are far less disruptive at home. Often they can be safely left in a different room.

Interruptions, especially the arrival of unexpected visitors, are a real problem in the community, and there is not much that can be done about it. Patients mostly sort these problems out for you, though some visitors will bowl in and want to know who you are, posing problems over confidentiality. You have to be prepared to improvise in these situations, and sometimes to abandon the interview altogether, to return at a later time.

Professional Boundaries

Maintaining boundaries is more difficult in the community. The psychiatrist's office offers an actual and a symbolic formality, which emphasises a distance between the doctor and the patient. Roles are more ambiguous in the home. Most patients offer you a cup of tea or coffee when you arrive, and participation in these ordinary social rituals is part of the process that makes for a different relationship. However, the offer (or, more importantly, the acceptance) of an alcoholic beverage clearly breaks a boundary. More subtly, it is easy for the relationship to shift towards something inappropriately reciprocal. You cannot help but behave in a more informal way in the community and this demands a constant awareness of professional boundaries.

Some patients, of course, tend to threaten boundaries because of the nature of their problem, for example some patients with borderline personality disorder who crave intimacy. Some types of patients cannot be visited at home appropriately by some types of professionals, for example male patients with a history of sexual aggression cannot be seen at home alone by female staff. These situations are another reason why there is always a need for residual clinic interviewing: there are no one-size-fits-all solutions.

Inefficiency

Few psychiatrists seem to doubt the superiority of home visits over clinic appointments, but some object that it is impractical to abandon clinics because home visiting is 'inefficient'.

They point out that they see a patient every 15 minutes in clinic, and that it is impossible to maintain this work rate if you add travelling time. On top of this, interviewing at home demands flexibility, as a second, or indeed third, visit may be needed to complete an assessment, whereas assessment can almost always be completed in a single one-hour appointment in the clinic.

What this fails to take into account is the alteration to team working and to the whole face of clinical practice that occurs when you move into the community. Where more than one team member is involved with a patient, follow-up visits can be conducted jointly, which saves time on meetings. Because it is easier to delay or cancel home visits than outpatient appointments, working practices are intrinsically more flexible. The better quality of home interviews means that they can occur less frequently. Letters can be dictated in the car between visits, which allows both team members to influence the content. Psychiatric clinics have high non-attendance rates, whereas the rate of failed home visits is far lower. This makes the use of time more efficient. Routine appointments can be reduced to periodic multidisciplinary reviews of treatment, perhaps only once a year. The internal dynamic of clinic booking systems leads inexorably to an autonomous rebooking cycle, which demands more frequent appointments.

Some psychiatrists concede that this style of practice is practical in cities, but object that it is impractical in rural settings where the population is more dispersed. In fact, in rural settings the majority of the population live together in settlements, and only a minority are widely dispersed. It might be that you cannot offer a true community service to very dispersed rural areas, but it is still possible to offer it to their neighbours in small towns and large villages.

Even if the objection that community psychiatry is prohibitively time consuming were true, it would not change the strongest argument for this style of working, which is that it works better, and that it is generally preferred by patients.

Dogs

Issues of safety are dealt with in Chapter 19, but no discussion of home interviewing would be complete without mentioning dogs. Unfortunately, the British are a nation of dog lovers, but there is a lamentable lack of canine reciprocation. Dogs are not, in general, a species of psychiatrist lovers. Ethology tells us that whilst dogs come in a wide variety of sizes, they are all territorial pack animals with a strong sense of hierarchy and conspicuous dentition. Dogs are a significant distraction in the clinical situation. Even when calm, certain breeds of dog, such as bull terriers, can present a surprisingly intimidating facial expression. Large dogs are not necessarily the biggest problem. Small dogs can be very aggressive, and are a particular problem for those of us who have lost line-of-sight contact with our shoes. Being bitten is not the only risk. Stepping on a pet is a poor prelude to a sensitive interview.

The point about dogs is that you need to know about them. It is worth asking about the presence of dogs within the household prior to visiting. Dog owners are rarely aware of the effect of their pet on visitors, and it is usually necessary to ask for them to be removed from the interview. It is sensible to have a method for flagging the clinical notes for the presence of dogs.

Psychiatric Emergencies in the Community

The concept of a psychiatric emergency is difficult, because mental illnesses tend to evolve relatively slowly, and quite often it is not the patient who thinks that there is an emergency.

There is an old adage that, in psychiatry, the term 'emergency' merely indicates that someone (patient, family member or professional) is frightened, and this is true. It is also true that emergencies often relate to factors other than changes in the patient's mental state. For example, 'emergencies' often arise on a Friday afternoon or before public holidays, because there is an anxiety that something bad will happen, not immediately, but before the next time help is readily available. Alternatively, emergencies can arise when the patient's mental state has shown little change, but someone new has suddenly become aware that they are unwell.

The essential components in resolving psychiatric emergencies in all settings are:

- to try to understand how the patient is experiencing the situation;
- to be clear who is in charge of managing the situation;
- to respond to the objective risks, not to speculative fears;
- to keep everybody's anxiety under control (including your own);
- to take the time that is needed to resolve the situation, rather than acting under external time pressure (for example, because a shift is ending). This often means retreating and taking time to think.

The good thing about attending an emergency situation in the community is that you can see for yourself what is happening, and you can gain a clear understanding of how the situation has developed. It may be possible to negotiate a treatment plan with the patient because you will be involved in delivering it. This can be decisive in avoiding compulsory admission.

Even if the patient was not frightened to begin with, he or she is likely to become so as an emergency assessment proceeds. Fear almost always makes a person's mental state deteriorate. The assessing psychiatrist is intruding into the patient's home and this can make people very angry. You have little control over the environment. There may well be frightened or distressed family members present. There may be ambulance staff, police officers, social workers, GPs and emergency vehicles. None of this will calm the patient down. At best, they will think they are likely to be admitted to hospital against their will. The patient is quite likely to put a paranoid interpretation on the situation. He or she will certainly notice if the situation is developing in an ominous way.

Planning is generally important, and this means collating as much information as possible before visiting the patient. When things go wrong during emergencies in the community, it can be distressing to learn later that an identical sequence of events occurred a few months earlier. If it is possible, you should speak to someone who knows the patient prior to visiting.

It is best to have a low-key initial visit before involving other services, though this is not always safe. Once you are in contact with the patient, it is a good principle to tell them what you intend to do at each stage. There is no role for misleading the patient or 'jumping' them, except under the most dangerous circumstances. Many patients, equipped with knowledge of your plans, will decide to go along with them.

The overall approach to interviewing and assessment needs to be heavily modified in emergency circumstances. There is little point in attempting to do a comprehensive assessment, as it is likely to be impossible and, in any case, background histories taken under such circumstances tend to be misleading. These are dynamic, evolving situations, and it is the decision-making process that is most important. You have often to make decisions without comprehensive information, on the basis of the balance of factors as the assessment proceeds. It is important to recognise that your decisions may prove to be less than optimal once full information is available. The strength of your conclusions should reflect the quality of the available evidence.

Some emergency interviews happen in public or semi-public places. Crowds can form, and strangers or neighbours can intervene. Some interviews are extremely fragmentary and are conducted, for example, whilst pursuing the patient through a busy shopping precinct. It can be difficult to maintain a proper professional persona and patient confidentiality. The personal dignity and safety of all involved can easily be compromised. You have to be prepared to give up if it is obvious that the assessment cannot be brought to a satisfactory conclusion.

Main Points in This Chapter

1. Community psychiatry involves psychiatrists working within a community rather than in a clinic.
2. Interviewing patients in their own home involves no new techniques, but does offer a new type of clinical information.
3. Working with patients in their own environment changes the therapeutic relationship and the nature of multidisciplinary working.
4. There are some difficulties in community interviewing, especially concerning confidentiality and maintenance of boundaries.
5. Psychiatric emergencies in the community are not easy to manage, but they benefit from planning and an awareness of the patient's perspective.

Fragmented Interviewing and Assessment

New Patterns of Psychiatric Practice

The last ten years have seen massive changes in the way that psychiatry is practised in the UK. To a lesser extent this has been evident in other countries as well, although some of the changes have brought UK practice more in line with patterns of care in some other European countries. The changes were never set out or announced as a plan or a policy initiative. There is no clarity as to the reasons why they have been adopted. Although there is variation between the countries that comprise the UK, in England the move away from long-standing patterns of care is now almost complete. The new pattern is known as functionalised care.

Over 70 years, the development of British psychiatry has been shaped by the existence of state-funded health and social care systems. The dominant pattern of care from the 1970s to the first decade of this century was integrated community care, whereby a single multi-disciplinary team offered patients a continuous relationship with specific individual practitioners. The relationship persisted through periods of inpatient and community treatment. This system had its faults, but it did have some real advantages in allowing teams to pursue consistent treatment strategies. It ensured that team members had a good knowledge of patients' backgrounds and their problems without the need for repeated assessments.

Functionalised care, on the other hand, involves amongst other things an entirely separate clinical team taking charge of care planning and delivery during inpatient stays. In the community, there are separate teams that provide specialised care during different phases of treatment, including crisis intervention/home treatment and early intervention teams, with some functions retained by generic CMHTs. Although older psychiatrists may lament the new pattern of care, this is the clinical environment in which we now work, and the challenges it presents must be met.

It is probably a reflection of the unplanned nature of the change that there is a paucity of guidance as to how assessment is supposed to work in the new system. There is guidance that says that patients do not like repetitive assessment and that this should be minimised, which is perfectly reasonable. What no one seems to know is how comprehensive and continuing assessment without repetition is supposed to be achieved. Box 15.1 describes a difficulty stemming from fragmented assessment.

The Challenges of Functionalised Care

Everyone agrees that comprehensive assessment is a prerequisite for good mental health care, including a good understanding of contextual factors beyond the patient's symptoms and

BOX 15.1 A Fragmentary Interview Goes Wrong

A 55-year-old man was admitted to a medical ward, having been brought to hospital by the police after they found him wandering and disorientated in an evident state of confusion. Investigations revealed no medical cause for his condition. On the ward, he was agitated, pacing on the spot and wringing his hands. He was slow to answer questions and he appeared preoccupied. He was not well orientated in time and place, and he was dependent on ward staff for basic self-care. He was referred to the general hospital liaison psychiatric team for assessment of possible dementia.

The liaison team mental health nurses spoke to his elderly parents, who were his nearest relatives. They explained that he had been working in a supermarket until six months earlier, when he had become increasingly gloomy about the future and started to think he had a terminal illness. He progressively neglected himself and stopped going to work. They had been taking hot meals to his flat for him daily, but he had stopped eating them.

The nurses arranged for an assessment on the medical ward by a consultant psychiatrist, and asked for the patient's parents to be present when he visited. The consultant was in a hurry between other appointments and attended alone, at a time when the nurses were busy. He read the medical case notes and interviewed the patient to assess his cognitive function. It was impaired. His assessment was that the patient had an early onset dementia and was likely to require residential care. He did not realise that the parents were present until he was ready to leave. He apologised to them and said that the nurses would explain his findings later.

The following day, nurses were concerned about the assessment, and asked a second psychiatrist to assess. She spoke with his parents and made a provisional diagnosis of depressive pseudo-dementia. Antidepressant medication was started, and four weeks later, the patient's cognitive state was normal.

immediate circumstances. Operational policies and guidance for specialist teams invariably emphasise the need for thorough assessment. There is usually an assumption that at some point patients will experience the kind of assessment that is described in the earlier chapters of this book, exemplified by a full office-based psychiatric assessment interview.

There is general acceptance that therapeutic outcomes are critically affected by the relationship between practitioner and patient, which is formed during assessment, as we have described. There is growing evidence on the importance of the therapeutic alliance and on the adverse consequences when the practitioner fails to achieve this.

The system of functionalised care makes these tasks challenging because it involves urgent interventions being broken down into at least three phases. There is likely to be an initial point of referral assessment, say in the emergency department, or in the patient's own home. There is likely to be a second assessment by the team offering immediate crisis care, say an acute inpatient team or a crisis resolution/home treatment team. When the patient has improved they are likely to be referred to another professional or team for follow-up, usually a psychiatrist or a CMHT.

In less urgent situations, there still are simple referrals to a psychiatrist who offers assessment and follow-up until the point of discharge in the traditional way. Often, however, people with less severe or acute problems move between primary care mental health teams (known as Improving Access to Psychological Therapies or IAPT teams in England) and CMHTs, or between consultant and other team members.

BOX 15.2 Obstructions to Good Quality Assessments and Successful Therapeutic Relationships in Functionalised Care

- Patients move between teams in a single episode of care.
- Interviews are conducted in less than ideal circumstances with a pressing need for immediate decisions.
- The system is impatient, with a high priority given to patient turnover at the expense of thorough assessment and therapeutic relationships.
- Assessments focus on current mental state at the expense of full contextual information.
- It is easy to overlook the absence of items of history where no one has responsibility for conducting a comprehensive assessment.
- Therapeutic relationships are hard to form because of the involvement of many different professionals. Undertakings made by one professional are easily broken by another professional.
- Information is easily lost as the patient crosses interfaces between teams.
- Communication between professionals is through the written word rather than discussion. This is not the optimal means of communication.

Shift working and changes of personnel can further complicate matters. It can be difficult for patients to understand or remember the specific roles of individual professionals they see, because the system is complicated and subject to regular reorganisation. Most clinicians correctly feel that there is no substitute for taking a history, or hearing the story, directly from the patient. The circumstances and the need to avoid excessive repetition can mean that everyone takes a partial, unsystematic history and yet feels that they 'know' the patient. It is a recipe for misunderstanding, lost information and inaccurate assessment unless active steps are taken to avoid this. Box 15.2 summarises the problems.

Managing Fragmentary Assessments

There is a good deal that can be done within organisations and within teams to ameliorate the difficulties caused by fragmented assessment processes. These measures are beyond the scope of this book, but needless to say, digital and paper records can be organised to make it easy to access previous assessments and to identify gaps. Few of us work with ideal record systems like this. The pace of change in services is too rapid for record systems to keep up with patterns of practice.

The first and most important point about fragmented assessments is that, when the patient is sitting in front of you, the template of a full history and the principles of forming a good therapeutic relationship have to remain in your awareness. Although it is in the nature of fragmented assessments that they involve cutting corners, this does not mean that the missing corners are of no consequence. You have an individual responsibility to do everything you can to ensure that a full assessment will eventually occur. We cannot avoid counsel of perfection: where the patient has had no previous contact with mental health services, as far as possible you should try to carry out a full assessment interview, even if this is not the expectation of the professionals around you. The more elements of a full assessment you miss out, the less reliable your conclusions will be. Doing things properly takes time, but it minimises the chance of error. Putting things right is much more time consuming than doing it right in the first place.

Many of the principles of interviewing with other team members set out in Chapter 12 are directly applicable to fragmented interviews, not least because these interviews are often conducted with other team members.

Preparation

As usual, it is important to be clear about the purpose of the interview and your role at the outset. This is not necessarily obvious. Assessments by functionalised teams do not always involve a psychiatrist, so why are you involved in this one? Are you there as a generic team member or to bring specific psychiatric expertise to the interview? Is the expectation that you will do a full assessment or just some element of the assessment? If the latter, who is going to do the elements you omit, and who is going to draw it together into a full assessment? If the answers to these questions are unclear, then you have little option but to carry out these tasks yourself.

In theory, the advent of digital record systems should have made it easy to access up-to-date information about the involvement of other mental health professionals with the patient. In practice, it takes time and effort to find and absorb the relevant information. Despite this, you should try to do so. You should read the notes yourself, in order to avoid risk diffusion, which is described below. It is particularly important to understand and record how you came to see this patient at this time, because the context of the assessment makes your findings more meaningful when someone else is looking at your notes some time later.

Conducting the Interview and Afterwards

In general, the more that a psychiatric interview feels like a normal conversation the better (without breaching professional boundaries), and the more that a fragmentary interview feels like a normal psychiatric interview the better. It is even more important than usual to ensure that the patient knows who you are by name, your professional role, why you are interviewing them, and how the outcome of this interview fits into their programme of assessment and care.

Although you may have no further contact with the patient, you should behave with the same attention to the therapeutic relationship as you would if you expected to deliver all of the treatment yourself. In fact, an off-hand, aloof or arrogant interview in the context of functionalised care can have a particularly destructive impact, because there may be no opportunity to put things right later. At best, the patient may come to feel that they are being taken less seriously by some teams or team members than others. At worst, they may reject the entire intervention.

If you have seen the patient before, you should acknowledge this, and tell them what you remember from the last interview. If there are gaps in your memory it is better to admit them at the outset, rather than have it become evident in the course of the interview, which is bound to undermine the patient's confidence in you. An honest acknowledgement of forgetfulness has a far less damaging effect, and may be experienced by the patient as an engaging admission of human fallibility.

Once the interview is drawing to a close, there is a particular pitfall when working in a functionalised care system, related to the fact that frequently you have no means of ensuring that what needs to happen next does occur in reality. From this point of view, fragmentary interviews are very different to the situation where you are able to take personal responsibility to ensure that appointments or visits will happen at the right time and that the direction that care follows will be on course.

Hard experience has demonstrated that multiple personnel and team interfaces create ample opportunity for things to go wrong. Consequently, it is a mistake to confidently tell the patient what is going to happen next, on the assumption that the various systems will function as expected or hoped. It is far better to tell patients what you think should happen, what you are going to do to make it happen and what they should do if it does not work out as you intend. It is particularly important on this last point to attend to detail. If you give a telephone number to call, you should be sure that it will not be permanently switched to voice mail. The patient should not be given contact details of someone who will tell them to go to see their GP to seek re-referral (a particularly disastrous thing to say to someone in crisis who has already tried to engage with a service). If a GP referral is the appropriate route to follow (which it rarely is) then it is best to tell the patient so from the outset, rather than setting in train a frustrating and fruitless telephone contact.

When fragmentary interviews are recorded, you should be careful to set out what you have omitted to do, particularly if you have failed to ask about significant areas of history. It is helpful to record who it is that you expect to fill the gaps and complete the assessment. A partial formulation is needed, because a decontextualised diagnosis is particularly misleading where you had no knowledge of some contextual factors in the first place. There is an implication in making a relatively unqualified diagnosis that nothing relevant has been omitted, but after a fragmentary interview leading to an incomplete assessment, you do not know if this is true or not.

Assessments that extend over more than one interview are discussed further in Chapter 16.

Risk Diffusion

Risk diffusion has always existed, but it is a particular problem in functionalised care systems. It is the term that we have coined to describe a process whereby no individual professional holds responsibility for assessing and managing the risk to a patient through an episode of care, so that concern over risk dissipates and important risk factors are overlooked.

In the worst case, a patient is passed from professional to professional and from team to team, and as the situation changes (or when the patient's symptoms and situation fail to improve), information is diluted and lost. Subtleties are overlooked, context is forgotten and hypothesising stops. In due course, decision-making is guided by little more than diagnosis, because detail has dropped away from the team's understanding of the patient and their situation. Diagnosis is never sufficient on its own to guide treatment planning or an understanding of risk.

The only real protection against risk diffusion is to be aware of it. It is particularly likely to arise as the patient is passed from one team to another. Face-to-face discussion is more effective than written handover, but even here it is possible for two professionals to persuade themselves that the risk is less severe than it really is, especially when neither of them knows the patient very well.

Main Points in This Chapter

1. Functionalised care can lead to the involvement of multiple professionals and teams during one episode of care.

2. This pattern of care does not relieve individual psychiatrists of the responsibility to make a full assessment wherever possible, and to be mindful of the continuing therapeutic relationship between the patient and the mental health service.

3. It is important to be clear in each interview what your role is, what parts of a full assessment have been omitted, and who is going to fill those gaps at a later stage. All of this should be communicated to the patient, and it should be clearly recorded.

4. You should not assume that complicated systems will work efficiently, because often they do not. Patients should have clear instructions about what to do when plans involving other professionals or teams are not carried out appropriately.

5. It is helpful to bear in mind risk diffusion, whereby responsibility for assessing and managing risk rests with no individual, and key information is lost in the patient's movement from one professional to another.

Chapter 16

'Impossible' Assessments

Psychiatrists sometimes confront clinical scenarios that they regard as 'impossible'. What makes these situations 'impossible', rather than 'difficult', is that the psychiatrist cannot make a full and reliable assessment of the patient, and yet they are expected to do so. The problem seems to have no solution. We consider two common examples: emergency assessment of intoxicated patients and the rhetorical interview. There are other scenarios, but making progress in the face of the 'impossible' rests on common principles, the most important of which is the willingness and ability to conduct an extended assessment over more than one interview.

Emergency Assessment of Intoxicated Patients

Alcohol and drug misuse are part of the fabric of modern life. In the UK, both are freely available and they are cheap. As we pointed out in Chapter 2, people with mental health problems have higher rates of substance misuse than the rest of the population, and substance misuse can be a cause of mental health problems. Intoxication releases disinhibited and alarming behaviour, and this can be the last straw for those caring for someone who is struggling with a mental health problem. It can lead to behaviour that attracts police attention. They often bring distressed, intoxicated people to emergency departments for assessment.

It is extremely difficult, if not impossible, to conduct a psychiatric interview with a drunken person, but huge amounts of conflict and anguish can result when mental health professionals refuse to try to do so. One reason for this is that it leaves some other department, agency or person with the difficult task of keeping the person safe until they are sober or sufficiently recovered to allow a meaningful interview to take place. Detailed guidance on the overall management of these situations is beyond the scope of this book, but it is available elsewhere (e.g. Poole 2015). We are interested here in applying principles to the assessment of people who are temporarily unable to participate fully.

Most psychiatrists are only too familiar with the dispiriting call to attend a general hospital emergency department where someone is threatening suicide and is intoxicated to the point of being drunk. Family or friends are often in attendance, insisting that the real problem is not alcohol but an underlying mental disorder. They correctly say that intoxication has exacerbated an existing problem and that alcohol is making the situation riskier. The patient is tearful and awkward, smells strongly of alcohol and is asking for something that cannot be agreed to, such as to be taken to a local multi-storey car park or similar dangerous place. The psychiatrist cannot have a meaningful conversation with the patient, who may well dismiss all suggestions of help as pointless, as they believe their situation to be beyond hope. Even when the patient is more amenable, it is difficult to place much faith in undertakings that he or she makes about short- or medium-term plans. The emergency department staff want the patient to go elsewhere, to make space for people with illnesses that they can treat, and mental health teams (whether hospital or community based) are very reluctant to accept responsibility for people who are intoxicated. In the meantime, the patient remains at risk.

Thresholds of Sobriety

Some mental health services have a policy that they will not assess anyone who is over the legal limit for driving. In the UK, this is a blood ethanol level of 80 mg/100 ml, which is rather high by international standards. Despite this, many people who are over this limit are not so intoxicated that interviewing them is pointless (although others will be very drunk, because of differences in alcohol tolerance). Breathalysers are invaluable in assessing whether a change in behaviour is due to rising intoxication, because alcohol is still being absorbed from stomach contents. They have no proper role in deciding whether someone is fit to be assessed.

The main features that would tend to suggest that a person cannot currently be assessed because of alcohol intoxication are aggressive behaviour; incomprehensible speech (including dysarthria and or a degree of repetition that allows no dialogue); ataxia; nystagmus; and sedation. It should be noted that some of these features are similar to those of Wernicke's encephalopathy (see below), which is a physical condition that requires urgent treatment.

Cooper and colleagues have suggested that where patients are intoxicated, the most meaningful test is whether the person has mental capacity to make decisions about their care and treatment (Cooper et al. 2010). Certainly, a face-to-face assessment has to be made in order to decide whether to proceed to a full clinical interview with someone who has been drinking or using drugs.

Extended Assessment versus Delayed Assessment

Even where a structured interview is inappropriate, it is usually possible to commence an extended assessment. This allows immediate decisions to be made on the basis of the best judgement that can be made at the time. The patient can be properly interviewed, and a full assessment made, once they have reached an appropriate level of sobriety.

Following first principles, history is the most important part of assessment. Relatives and other informants are likely to be able to give a good deal of relevant information. The patient's GP may well have useful information. The local alcohol team may know the patient. In the case of people who are repeated attenders at emergency departments, there may be a lot of information that can be gleaned from medical notes. There is a risk that informants either collude through minimisation or exaggerate in desperation. This under-lines the importance of gaining information from more than one source. When history is gathered primarily from informants, it is helpful to focus on recent events. The accounts are likely to be more accurate about what has happened in the immediate past and, in any case, these are key to immediate concerns. The major exception is that it is essential to find out how the person has behaved in the past under similar circumstances, no matter how long ago the last occasion might have been. A person who has recently returned to drinking after two decades of total abstinence is very likely to show a return to behaviour that has been absent for a very long time.

In order to make appropriate assessments of intoxicated people, there have to be organisational systems and agreements that work. Emergency departments must be prepared to look after the patient until they are fit for interview. They will normally accept this if it is accompanied by the quid pro quo that the patient will be fully assessed promptly on becoming sober. Patient and staff safety has to be actively managed in the interim.

Key Objectives in a Partial Assessment

Some of the key objectives of a partial assessment are, strictly speaking, somebody else's job. For example, in most emergency departments, an emergency physician is meant to exclude physical disorder prior to referral to a psychiatrist. However, we live in an imperfect world, and these assessments are sometimes less than thorough. More importantly, a key reason that psychiatrists are medically qualified is that they are the experts on the behavioural presentation of organic disorder. The assessing psychiatrist has to make his or her own mind up whether this is present. This is not only on first assessment; the possibility of physical disorder must be borne in mind throughout treatment.

- The first and most important objective is to gather sufficient information to exclude the possibility that there is organic pathology that requires immediate treatment. This includes injuries or acute biological events, which may or may not be due to intoxication. A broken limb due to a fall can easily go unnoticed if the person's behaviour is distractingly disorganised due to intoxication. A myocardial infarction may not present in the usual way in someone who is seriously drunk.
- The second objective is to ensure that the person's disordered behaviour really is due to intoxication. Acute and chronic heavy drinking has some medical consequences that mimic or exacerbate the confusion caused by intoxication. When people who are drunk fall over, they do not put their hands out quickly enough to protect their heads. This accounts for the association between drinking and subdural haemorrhage, at least in part. Subdural haemorrhage can present without localising signs, but with a picture very like drunkenness. The onset of symptoms may be delayed for days after the initial fall. Wernicke's encephalopathy, characterised by ataxia, confusion and ophthalmoplegia (see below) can present like intoxication. It is due to acute thiamine deficiency, which can be provoked by the glucose load in a proper meal eaten after arrival at hospital. Conversely, Wernicke's may present with a fall at home. People with alcohol problems are at risk of cirrhosis and acute liver failure, and both can lead to hepatic encephalopathy. It is important to recognise that this is not always immediately accompanied by clinically obvious jaundice.
- The next objective is to assess risk to self and others. This subject is dealt with more fully in Chapter 19. We emphasise that proper risk assessment can only be made on the basis of full information and careful clinical assessment, but sometimes you just have to make a judgement on the basis of inadequate evidence. In the case of intoxication, there are three particular questions:
  - . To what extent does the risk primarily relate to acute intoxication?
  - . To what extent does the risk relate to an underlying problem that is not related to substance misuse per se?

. Where the risk is associated with intoxication, how likely is this to recur, how quickly, and who is likely to be around when it does?
• The final objective is to form an explicit hypothesis, with clarity about the factors that lead you to this conclusion. In the event that the person's condition does not progress or develop as you expect, an explicit hypothesis helps you to recognise this, and avoids a rigid and inappropriate attachment to misleading first impressions.

Specific High Risk Presentations

There are a handful of specific circumstances that can arise with, or be mistaken for, acute alcohol intoxication that assessing psychiatrists need to watch out for, because they carry particular risks to the patient. These are: intoxication with more than one substance; Wernicke's encephalopathy; and alcohol withdrawal.

Alcohol/Drug Combinations

The penetration of drug use into the mainstream of life means that people who have taken an excess of alcohol have often taken other psychoactive substances as well. This is true of all age groups and includes both illicit and prescribed drugs. The presentation of combined intoxication is extremely variable, and there is no way of working out what substances are causing what from the patient's clinical presentation. You have to find out, if you can, from the patient or from informants what they have taken. The effects do not always pass quickly, and two particular combinations are especially dangerous.

The first is alcohol and other sedative drugs, especially opioids. These substances cause depression of respiratory drive alone and synergistically. The combination is a common cause of death, usually (though not always) following aspiration of stomach contents. Drugs and alcohol are absorbed at different rates, so that the time of highest risk may arise long after the patient arrives for assessment. If a patient has been noisy and aggressive earlier on, it is understandable that health professionals are tempted to leave well alone when they go quiet. If they snore loudly, this is not a sign of sleeping soundly; it is a sign of respiratory distress. When patients become unrousable, intervention is needed.

The second is alcohol and stimulants, especially cocaine. Heavy acute use of cocaine is a potent cause of stroke, and alcohol exacerbates the risk. The mechanism is uncertain, but transient hypertension is plausible. Blood pressure should be measured wherever possible when the patient is intoxicated, but especially where stimulants have also been taken. The combination can also induce confusion, fearfulness, hallucinations, paranoia and, sometimes, suicidal despair.

A final point about intoxication, whether due to single or combined substances, is that presentations of disturbed behaviour that persist for more than 24 hours are likely to be due either to an underlying cause other than intoxication, or a complication, such as the toxic psychosis that can arise after large doses of amphetamine, which may persist for several days. We continue to counsel extreme caution over the use of the diagnosis 'drug induced psychosis' (Komuravelli et al. 2011), which has little or no explanatory power.

Wernicke's Encephalopathy

This disorder, which is an acute manifestation of Vitamin B1 (thiamine) deficiency, has become increasingly common in recent years. As mentioned above, arrival at and admission to hospital are particular high risk times for it to emerge *de novo*. It is not easy to develop thiamine deficiency if you consume a typical Western diet. It is a condition that tends to affect middle-aged people who have been heavy drinkers for many years, and who neglect themselves. People like this develop thiamine deficiency for two main reasons. Heavy drinkers eat badly, because they lose their appetite and prioritise alcohol consumption. Their calorific intake comes mainly from ethanol and sugar in drinks. Most of the thiamine in our diet comes from vegetables, grains and fruit. Alcohol and potato crisps constitute a very low thiamine diet. Secondly, high levels of alcohol inhibit thiamine absorption, so that what little thiamine is consumed, for example, in yeast cells in beer, is poorly absorbed.

Thiamine is stored in the liver, but it is used up during glucose metabolism. Consequently, people who have incipient thiamine deficiency can be precipitated into Wernicke's encephalopathy after a few cheese sandwiches, offered in hospital as a humane response to their evident malnourishment. If Wernicke's encephalopathy is not treated vigorously with intravenous thiamine, it is likely to proceed to a permanent brain injury in the form of Korsakoff's syndrome, characterised by profound short-term memory impairment.

The main features of Wernicke's encephalopathy are confusion, memory impairment, ataxia, ophthalmoplegia and nystagmus. Older doctors, such as us, were taught that there was a triad of symptoms: confusion, ophthalmoplegia and ataxia. However, all three elements are rarely present, as eye signs are not very common. Impaired consciousness with marked ataxia is the most frequent presentation.

Alcohol Withdrawal

Alcohol withdrawal is a consequence of tolerance to alcohol. Tolerance is predominantly a neuronal phenomenon and not, as is often supposed, a result of liver enzyme induction. Alcohol suppresses neuronal membrane activity and has marked anticonvulsant effects. When neurones operate in an environment with continuous high levels of alcohol, membrane excitability is up-regulated as a homeostatic adjustment. When alcohol abruptly disappears from the body, the neurones are left in a state of hyper-excitability, which causes the symptoms of acute withdrawal. These can progress to delirium tremens (DTs) and epileptic seizures. The latter, in turn, can cause status epilepticus and death. Withdrawal seizures can occur in the absence of DTs. Needless to say, acute alcohol withdrawal is a potentially life-threatening, but fully treatable, condition.

The features of alcohol withdrawal short of DTs are restlessness, over-arousal, anxiety, 'jitteriness', tremor and sleep disturbance. When DTs occurs, these features are more severe, accompanied by fluctuations in consciousness, paranoid ideas, severe fearfulness, auditory and visual hallucinations, irritability and aggression. There is often a key feature, which is common whenever hallucinations have an organic origin, of marked behavioural responses, such as flinching, cowering or shouting back.

People who are in alcohol withdrawal act oddly, and often smell similar to people who are intoxicated. Taken together with a history of heavy drinking and having the appearance of being an 'alcoholic', this can lead to an error whereby someone who is in alcohol withdrawal and in need of immediate treatment is thought to be drunk.

Interviewing Intoxicated People

Although interviewing people when they are intoxicated may not be very fruitful from the point of view of assessment of their mental state, it still has to be done. It is not sensible to try to conduct the interview alone. The interview should be conducted by two health professionals working together. They need to agree beforehand who will lead the interview, and what they will do if the patient becomes aggressive. It is never helpful to try to assess a patient if you feel frightened, as it invites mistakes and errors of judgement. Bravado places the doctor and the patient at risk.

An appropriate environment makes a big difference to these interviews, but the vast majority of them are conducted in suboptimal conditions. A quiet, comfortable, well-lit environment without a lot of extraneous noise, attended by calm and sympathetic staff is perfect, but exceedingly rare. There are some factors that the interviewer has control over. Politeness and clarity about what is happening, what you want, and what is likely to happen next, together with a willingness to repeat all of this a few times without becoming noticeably irritated, can make a surprisingly big difference to the success of the interview, and in the patient's behavioural response to it.

There are some questions of immediate importance that only the patient can answer. Prominent amongst these is what they have drunk and what other substances they have taken in the past 24 hours. Quantities alone are insufficient information. You also need to know how quickly it has been consumed. A bottle of vodka consumed over a whole day will make the person noticeably intoxicated. The same quantity consumed over an hour and a half is likely to prove lethal.

The Rhetorical Interview

The rhetorical interview is not a new phenomenon, but it seems to have become far more frequent. The term does not refer to the common situation in everyday clinical practice where the patient or someone else has a particular diagnosis or outcome in mind from the outset. This is inevitable and it does not necessarily cause major problems in conducting an assessment. There is far more difficulty when the patient (or someone very close to them) has a strong emotional investment in a particular diagnosis or outcome to such an extent that they tailor their responses to guide you in the right direction. They become alarmed or angry if you appear to be moving away from the desired destination. This is the rhetorical interview proper, where at least one party regards the process as an argument to be won, rather than an exercise in collaborative understanding.

If rhetorical interviews really are becoming more common, it is probably due to a few easily identified factors. The general public are much better informed about the nature and treatment of mental illness and other mental health problems than they used to be, and they can access a certain amount of information, and huge amounts of disinformation, through the Internet. We are living through difficult times, including seemingly interminable austerity for public services and welfare benefits. People who are chronically unwell, or who find themselves at the bottom end of the social scale for other reasons, have much harder lives than they did previously. There are far fewer resources to assist them. It is hardly surprising that people sometimes feel that a formal psychiatric diagnosis might confer some advantages to them, notwithstanding the stigma that is attached to the labels. This is not to suggest that significant numbers of people seek a diagnosis when they are aware that there is nothing wrong with them, although a small number do. It is more the case that a specific psychiatric label can appear helpful to people who are living on the margins of society.

> **BOX 16.1** Rhetorical Interviews
>
> - Diagnostic (e.g. 'I've got bipolar disorder', 'He's got Asperger's Syndrome')
> - Specific treatments (e.g. 'I've got ADHD and I need methylphenidate')
> - Criminal charges ('I wasn't shoplifting, it was an automatism due to the diazepam')
> - Employment ('My employer shouted a lot, and now I've got PTSD')
> - Child contact ('I need a report saying that I'm only violent to adults')
> - Benefits ('They are taking my benefits off me and I've been advised to get my depression properly diagnosed')
> - Aetiology (organic) ('They think it's all in my mind, but it's neurological')
> - Aetiology (victimisation) ('The only reason I act in this way is because I was abused as a child')

Types of Rhetorical Interview

The content of these interviews can be very varied, but they mostly follow a few themes. The most common are set out in Box 16.1. These are not mutually exclusive. It is immediately obvious that in each of these scenarios, the patient (or relative) may be right. The rhetorical element is the determination to achieve a particular outcome by trying firmly to steer the interview in that direction.

For example, unstable mood is common, but it is not necessarily a symptom of mental disorder per se. Widespread publicity about bipolar disorder (not in itself a bad thing), together with the promotion by some researchers and clinicians of a proliferation of subtypes involving forme fruste symptoms (diagnoses which are not necessarily recognised or accepted by the majority of clinicians in the UK) has driven significant numbers of people to seek assessment in the belief that they have this condition. Some of them do have bipolar disorder, but many do not. An increased rate of detection might be a good thing, but some people with chronic social and emotional difficulties attend appointments with psychiatrists in the forlorn hope that a diagnosis of bipolar affective disorder will bring understanding and solutions. Similarly, publicity about autistic spectrum disorders and attention deficit hyperactivity disorder (ADHD) has led a significant group of people to seek assessment, usually for their male offspring or partner.

In rhetorical interviews, the person concerned has already made up their mind about the diagnosis; they do not wonder if that is the problem, they are certain that it is, and that many of their problems will be resolved if the diagnosis is made 'official'. As a psychiatrist, if you cannot explore other possibilities, then you cannot make the diagnosis properly, even when the patient or relative is right. The situation is highly dysfunctional from the outset, because the interview cannot go well, irrespective of the true nature of the problem.

The rhetorical search for a specific treatment sometimes involves a medication that is controversial for one reason or another. The use of stimulants for ADHD symptoms in adults is one such treatment, as there are no generally accepted criteria for their use. It is hard to agree to prescribe these drugs when, for example, the patient tells you that they only got through their PhD because they used illicit amphetamine. Requests for cannabis or cannabis derivatives are also common, probably because of the intense interest on the Internet in the therapeutic potential of the drug. A proportion of the general population believes that cannabis is benign in comparison with synthetic drugs because it is 'natural'.

The most common request with regard to cannabis is that it should be prescribed for pain, but it is sometimes requested for epilepsy. The request is sometimes for a 'get-out-of-jail-free' card in the form of a letter from the doctor saying that the patient has been advised to purchase cannabis on the black market for medicinal purposes.

Psychiatric assessment in pursuit of legal proceedings, or in order to secure a pension or welfare benefits, is sometimes more closely linked to a desire to press for confirmation of a particular level of disability or impairment rather than a specific diagnosis. This can involve significant exaggeration (although when a third party has initiated the referral, there may be a converse denial of impairment by the patient). This is especially difficult in the situation where someone is in danger of not being awarded, or losing, welfare benefits. At present in the UK large numbers of significantly disabled people are having welfare payments withdrawn and being told that they are fit for work. To a clinician, many of them do not appear to be fit for work at all, and they often become distressed about their situation. It can be impossible to assess the degree of underlying depression under these circumstances, even where the interview is not rhetorical. Understandable reactions to the prospect of impoverishment cannot always be distinguished from underlying problems. The interview is further complicated by an ethical dilemma. If you take the line of least resistance and simply do as the patient asks without independently satisfying yourself of the facts, then everyone is happy in the short run. In the long run, your ability to challenge perverse decisions is undermined, because benefit assessors are vigilant for the 'soft-touch' supporting clinician.

Yet another scenario involves a patient with a chronic condition who wants you to exclude the possibility that any psychological factor is relevant to their condition. There always are major psychological aspects to chronic illnesses, including diabetes, heart failure and hypertension. This is closely related to a converse but equally untenable situation. This is where someone tries to argue that they are too psychologically damaged to be considered an active agent in their own life, and seeks to be absolved of all personal responsibility for their own actions.

All in all, rhetorical interviews seem to create insurmountable obstacles to proper assessment. Nevertheless the psychiatrist still has the responsibility to try to undertake one.

Understanding Rhetorical Interviews

The likelihood of a rhetorical interview may be evident during the referral process. The patient or family are exasperated before they even meet you, and the referral letter makes it clear that you are expected to act as a court of appeal in an existing disagreement. Sometimes the patient or family set out their rhetorical case at the beginning of the interview. The most difficult rhetorical interviews are not immediately obvious, and the rhetorical agenda becomes evident slowly or late in the assessment. It is helpful to refer back to the principles we set out in the Introduction to this book, which are reiterated in Box 16.2.

In the overwhelming majority of cases, the patient and/or family are sincere in their belief about the importance of a particular outcome. However, dishonest people do exist, and there may be an element of deliberate falsehood. We deal with the issue of patients who lie in Chapter 8. Nothing in psychiatry is ever entirely simple; needless to say, dishonesty is not incompatible with the presence of a mental health problem.

In Chapter 8 we explored the problem of situations where the doctor and the patient hold conflicting agendas that are difficult to reconcile. We also explored the concept of the

> **BOX 16.2** Five Principles of Interviewing
>
> - Process: interviewing is an interaction that has a beginning, middle and end.
> - Patient-centredness: understanding and addressing the patient's concerns by attempting to resolve the doctor's and the patient's agendas.
> - Context: the patient's psychological and social context, the purpose of the interview and the professional's psychological and social background are important.
> - Hypothesising: skilled clinicians operate by forming hypotheses and testing them. Conscious awareness of the hypothesising process is helpful.
> - Clinical scepticism: a critical and independent-minded quality that questions psychiatric orthodoxy and recognises that all clinical information arrives through a lens of subjectivity.

meta-agenda, a set of background attitudes and beliefs that have an unhelpful impact on the interview. There is a meta-agenda that links nearly all rhetorical interviews:

Something is being withheld from me that is my entitlement

and

Nothing will come right for me unless I can secure that which is being withheld

These patients and/or families are angry from the outset. Their anger may be immediately evident if you are experienced as a representative of a profession that is complicit in their problem. Alternatively you may be seen as a potential ally until you start to disrupt the rhetorical agenda. Either way, conflict is extremely hard to avoid, even where you think that the patient is right about the diagnosis or treatment. Appropriate clinical scepticism, which is necessary in making a proper assessment, is likely to provoke a reaction of frustration and hostile helplessness based upon previous disappointments and rejections.

Any conflict in the room is likely to be focused on whether you believe or trust the patient's account; whether you are conducting your assessment properly; and whether you are influenced by some previous authority, usually another doctor. Disagreement or scepticism is taken as an attack on the authenticity of the patient's account of their suffering.

The doctor does appear to be in a no-win situation. The patient, or those close to them, will only be satisfied by a specific outcome. They have an argument that they want to make in support of that outcome. They will resist being deflected.

Managing Rhetorical Interviews

Box 16.3 summarises some important points in managing rhetorical interviews.

As it usually is possible to anticipate a rhetorical interview, it can be helpful to have a pre-assessment discussion with the referrer. This allows you to understand what has gone before and what the patient is likely to want. You may be able to work out what is likely to happen in the interview and to plan how you will proceed.

Patients often bring family or friends with them to these interviews as back-up. It can be difficult to insist on seeing the patient alone. If you cannot achieve this, the chances of a successful outcome are minimal. The interview will be hard to control, anger will feed around the room and negotiation will be more or less impossible. It is worth fighting for an initial one-to-one interview. The exception is that a trained mental health advocate can be incredibly helpful. A trained advocate will make sure that the patient's concerns are

BOX 16.3 Managing Rhetorical Interviews

1. If a rhetorical interview seems likely, have a discussion with the referrer in order to anticipate what might happen.
2. Plan the interview, if necessary extending assessment over two sessions before it is completed.
3. Try to interview the patient alone if you possibly can.
4. Acknowledge the rhetorical agenda early on, and let the patient talk about this, but also explain the difficulties that this causes for you.
5. If anger dominates the interview, say why this is a problem and try to get the patient to take responsibility for using the interview constructively.
6. Delay making a judgement where necessary, but always tell the patient the outcome face to face.
7. Document the reasons for your opinions carefully and send a copy of your report to the patient.
8. Accept that none of the above may work, and that things may go wrong later.

addressed without derailing the interview. Their supportive presence is likely to make the patient feel more relaxed. They will remember what you have said more clearly than the patient will.

Once the patient is in the room, it is helpful to acknowledge the rhetorical issue early on (as discussed in Chapter 8). You have to allow the patient to ventilate their sense of frustration and anger. They will make their case, which can allow a wider exploration in the second half of the interview. It creates an opportunity for the doctor to explain their dilemma, including the need to make up their own mind. Occasionally, this insistence on independent-mindedness infuriates the patient, and brings the interview to a premature end. The only consolation in this eventuality is that it is unlikely that any other strategy would have been more successful.

Fortunately, sudden and catastrophic ends to rhetorical interviews are uncommon, but some expression of anger is invariable. Even a controlled expression of anger can become seriously counterproductive if it continues for very long. It is easy for people to get into a spiral of indignant anger when you fail to agree with them. As in all psychiatric interviews, it is important to remain calm and reasonable, and to make sure that whatever you say will withstand repetition in other forums, as complaints after these interviews are common. If necessary, it can be helpful to state explicitly that the interview is turning into an angry rant, that time is limited, and that the patient might want to use the time differently.

Whatever happens, you can only complete an assessment if the patient will allow you to probe, challenge and identify gaps in history in the normal way. How you do this depends very much on the time available to you. An extended assessment is one way of achieving this. In the first interview you allow the patient to express their sense of grievance and make their case, trying to establish your credibility as someone who will listen. The actual assessment takes place in a second, calmer, interview. The second interview should take place quite soon after the first, no more than a week or two later. This may be difficult to arrange in modern NHS practice, but it is the approach that is most likely to help you get past the rhetorical agenda.

Rhetorical interviews can be exhausting for the patient and the psychiatrist alike. It is usually wise to avoid discussing your conclusions hurriedly at the end of a difficult interview. Calm reflection improves clinical judgement. However, no matter how unwelcome your conclusions are likely to be, they will be less destructive if they are delivered face to face. The temptation to avoid unpleasantness has to be resisted, because it will only confirm beliefs that the medical profession are unbending, monolithic and ungiving. If you fail to deliver the desired outcome for the patient, there is a strong possibility that there will be an 'I forgot to tell you that …' moment. This may demand further thought about the new information.

After the interview, a full and careful report that clearly sets out the reasons for your opinions is essential. It should be copied to the patient.

In our experience, it is possible to achieve a reasonably successful outcome for the patient in a significant proportion of these situations. No matter what you do, many of these clinical encounters end unhappily, and even where things go well at first, they are quite likely to go wrong later.

Main Points in This Chapter

1. Some, but not all, seemingly impossible obstacles to appropriate assessment can be overcome.
2. The best guide to deciding whether to assess a person who is intoxicated is their ability to participate in the interview rather than a particular threshold level of intoxication.
3. Life-threatening physical problems are easily overlooked in people who are intoxicated (or who appear to be intoxicated), such as Wernicke's encephalopathy, delirium tremens and subdural haemorrhage.
4. Rhetorical interviews occur where the patient tries to lead you to a predetermined conclusion, and becomes distressed when you explore other possibilities.
5. The fact that the patient or carers approach the interview as a rhetorical exercise does not necessarily mean that they are wrong.
6. Understanding the meta-agenda of rhetorical interviews is helpful. This usually involves the perception of an entitlement withheld and a belief that securing that entitlement is the only solution to the problem.
7. When an assessment looks impossible, extending it over two or more interviews can be helpful.

Developmental assessment is a specialist skill in child psychiatry and in the assessment of intellectual disability, but all psychiatrists must be able to bring a developmental perspective to their work. People with disorders that are believed to have a neurodevelopmental origin are routinely seen in non-specialist settings. Personality is best understood from a developmental point of view.

All psychiatrists must be able to raise the possibility of a developmental disorder on the basis of a careful and systematic assessment. It may not be appropriate for them to make a definitive diagnosis of these disorders, as this takes time. Some of these diagnoses have far-reaching consequences and they must be made with care. Nonetheless, if you are unable to feel confident in exploring developmental disorders, it is impossible to distinguish them from other psychiatric diagnoses.

Chapter 17

Neurodevelopmental Assessment

At primary school, another pupil puzzled Simon Perry. James White was odd. James was clumsy, slow and awkward. He had a peculiar and formal way of talking. He did not make eye contact. He was solitary and repetitive in his play. He would become preoccupied with tiny minutiae of everyday life. Simon Perry had a duffel bag that could be locked. James White made up a song about it: 'Simon Perry's got the key to his duffel bag, key to his duffel bag, key to his duffel bag.' He could be seen in his corner of the playground at break time, singing the song whilst dancing from foot to foot and flapping his hands. James became distressed very easily if teased, but he coped with his schoolwork. He was by far the best pupil in the whole school at mathematics. His speed and accuracy at mental arithmetic were astonishing. Some of the children said his mother had fallen down the stairs of a double-decker bus when she was pregnant, and that that explained his peculiarities.

In the 1970s, Simon Perry was a medical student on placement at a large mental hospital. There was a female patient from one of the long-stay wards whom he noticed striding purposefully around the hospital. Although she was evidently in her late thirties, she wore her hair in bunches and clutched a doll under her arm. One morning, she strode up to him and demanded to know his name and date of birth. He told her. She immediately snapped back 'You were born on a Friday' and stormed off. She was right. After that, every time she spotted him, she rushed over and said 'Your name is Simon Perry and you were born on Friday 25th November 1955.' Eventually he asked the staff about her. They told him that she was diagnosed with chronic schizophrenia. He was perplexed, because he could not see how that diagnosis explained her behaviour.

The details have been altered, but the above is essentially true. Early curiosity about James White and the woman with the doll was a factor that led Simon Perry to become a psychiatrist with an interest in neurodevelopmental disorders.

Making a firm diagnosis of a neurodevelopmental disorder should be done with care. Like the diagnosis of personality disorder, a neurodevelopmental diagnosis can be difficult to undo. All psychiatrists need some skills related to neurodevelopmental assessment, because people with significant problems often go without assessment or diagnosis in childhood, and are later referred to mental health services. Although psychiatric interest in autism spectrum disorder (ASD) and ADHD has grown, there are continuing problems with over-diagnosis, failure to diagnose and misidentification of the different neurodevelopmental disorders.

Mild to moderate intellectual disability (learning disability) is common amongst people seen by general adult psychiatrists. There is rising public awareness of ASD and ADHD, with an increasing demand for assessment for these conditions. Tourette's syndrome attracts less publicity, but it is relatively common. People with multiple tic disorder can present to a wide range of different services. We will outline the general principles of non-specialist assessment of neurodevelopmental disorder in adults, and briefly consider specific issues in making a primary assessment for each of the four major diagnoses that are likely to present to general psychiatrists. It is important to understand the syndromes, and to recognise that they overlap with each other.

General Principles of Neurodevelopmental Assessment

The first thing to understand about neurodevelopmental problems is that they are not categorical in nature. They are dimensional, so that there is no clear line of demarcation between 'normality' (or 'neurotypicality') and frank disorder. This is true of many other conditions seen by psychiatrists, especially personality disorder. It is equally true of many disorders affecting organ systems other than the brain. Although neurodevelopmental disorders cannot be regarded as diseases or illnesses, it does not follow that they can be dismissed as mere social constructs for the marginalisation of 'deviance'. They are associated with increased risk for symptoms of other psychiatric disorders, such as anxiety, depression, OCD and psychosis.

When severe, these problems can be distressing, with major consequences for every aspect of the person's life, although other people's reactions to unusual behaviour are a substantial part of what makes life difficult. There is an element of inference in the statement that they have their origins in the development of the neural substrate, with stronger evidence for this in some disorders than others. The question of what 'causes' these disorders is somewhat abstract, as they all have major psychological and social aspects that are just as important as biological atypicality.

It is generally possible for a non-specialist psychiatrist to exclude a neurodevelopmental problem, or to make a diagnosis in the presence of clear manifestations and an unambiguous neurodevelopmental history. In cases of ambiguity, it is necessary to secure a specialist opinion. The continuity with neurotypicality means that it is particularly important to record the severity of specific features in terms of their impact on everyday life, so that it is later possible to understand why you reached your conclusions. You may have access to the accounts of parents and other informants who will not be available to later clinicians. Box 17.1 sets out the main headings for a neurodevelopmental assessment.

BOX 17.1 Elements of Neurodevelopment History

- General psychiatric assessment
- Seek contemporaneous sources of information
- Family history of problems with language, learning and social relationships
- Milestones
- Speech and language
- Motor skills
- Friendships and peer relationships
- Play and interests
- Learning and education
- Changes/continuity through adolescence and adult life

Although these disorders should be evident from early childhood, many people do not receive an assessment or diagnosis until adulthood. For example, it is not uncommon for children to struggle throughout their schooling without formal testing, as the problems are attributed to laziness, conduct disorder or deviant attitudes to education within the family. On psychometric testing as adolescents or adults, it is common for people who have performed badly in mainstream schooling to have an assessed IQ well below 70.

General Psychiatric Assessment

Assessment of neurodevelopmental disorders does not stand alone, as a separate process. It occurs in the context of a general psychiatric assessment as described in Section 1 of this book. History taking and, to a lesser extent, mental state examination will elicit a large proportion of the information you need. The specific and detailed neurodevelopmental part of the assessment should be integrated with the usual interviewing schemata, so that it flows naturally from the topic headings that you always have in mind. Ordinary clinical curiosity helps you to explore and to understand the exact nature and consequences of the current problems that are provoking a suspicion of neurodevelopmental disorder.

Contemporaneous Sources of Information

Whilst the patient's own account is important, there will be some questions that they cannot answer. If they can, their answers will be based on what they have been told by parents or others who cared for them as a child. Contemporaneous sources of information are invaluable, especially if there is more than one source. Where you cannot interview adults who were around at the time, you have to be cautious about conclusions. The accounts of siblings (especially if older) and information in old school reports can be useful.

Family History

In addition to the usual family history enquiry, you should ask about individuals in the extended family who have had problems with language, learning and social relationships.

Developmental Milestones

Were walking, talking, daytime continence or reading delayed? If so, what happened? For example, did the child communicate non-verbally? Or shuffle on their backside instead of walking?

Speech and Language

Were there any unusual features of early and later speech, such as idiosyncratic use of vocabulary or incorrect use of pronouns? Were there problems in the articulation or clarity of speech? Did they ever see a speech or language therapist? Do they have a tendency to take things that people say too literally? Do they understand verbal humour?

Motor Skills

You should enquire about clumsiness, balance and dexterity, and whether problems improved with time. Skills with a ball, drawing, handwriting and in using cutlery can give a good indication of fine motor skills. Some people who have a general problem with fine motor skills have a particular skill in one area, for example drawing or playing a musical instrument. On enquiry, it often turns out that this skill has been developed through a strong interest and extended effort.

Friendships and Peer Relationships

Did they form friendships easily or with difficulty? How many friends did they have? What kind of child did they form friendships with, and what was the quality of relationships? Did they have a special friend? Were they bullied? Did they bully others? Did they have imaginary friends, and if so, how long did they persist (persistent imaginary friends are common in ASD)?

Play and Interests

Since the mid-1990s, even very young children have used digital devices for play, so that it may be necessary to ask carefully what games and social media the patient preferred, and how much time was devoted to them. Current usage is also relevant. The repertoire of play is important, as is the age at which imaginative and imitative play emerged. Are interests diverse and transient or narrow and intense? If the patient seems solitary, is this a preference or a consequence of social avoidance?

Learning

Ask about academic progress and attainment, and about conduct at school. Did they ever require support in learning at school, for example with literacy or numeracy? Far more children receive episodes of targeted support than ever go through a formal assessment of their educational needs.

Changes/Continuity

If changes have occurred, what are they? Are current problems and patterns of behaviour continuous with childhood difficulties? Did earlier problems improve/resolve? Disorders that manifest themselves for the first time in adulthood are highly unlikely to be developmental in origin. Where adult onset is described, look for evidence of earlier related problems, in other words for evidence that the disorder is not new, but has changed in manifestation.

Intellectual Disability (Learning Disability)

This involves an impairment of intellectual function that is evident from early life and which is accompanied by problems in social and adaptive behaviour. In Western Europe, 1 per cent of children have cognitive impairment. About 10 per cent of the population have an intellectual or specific learning disability (most commonly dyslexia) of a degree that affects their daily social functioning. More men are affected than women (this gender difference is apparent in all neurodevelopmental disorders, the disparity being greatest in ASD).

There are a number of specific causes of intellectual disability, such as Down syndrome, Fragile X syndrome, foetal alcohol syndrome and foetal rubella infection, but much intellectual disability does not involve a specific syndrome. Childhood environment and other social and psychological factors can significantly exacerbate intellectual disability.

The definitions in the classification systems are useful in identifying the features that assessment should focus on.

ICD-10 emphasises the vulnerability of people with intellectual disability (referred to as 'mental retardation' by the WHO). In particular, it points out that people with 'mental retardation' have three to four times higher prevalence of other mental disorders than the general population, and an increased risk of exploitation and physical or sexual abuse. ICD-10 points out that mild 'mental retardation' may not be evident unless the person is removed from their normal supportive social environment.

DSM-5 draws out specific deficits:

Deficits of Intellectual Functioning

- Reasoning
- Problem solving
- Planning
- Abstract thinking
- Judgement
- Academic learning
- Experiential learning

Deficits of Adaptive Functioning

- Communication
- Social skills
- Personal independence at home or in the community
- School or occupational functioning

The problems caused by intellectual disability tend to get worse as a child grows older and is exposed to more demanding social environments. Mild generalised cognitive impairment may not be obvious until the child starts attending school.

Psychometric testing of intellectual ability is outside of the scope of non-specialist assessment. Although the concept has been subject to criticism for a very long time, IQ testing using the Wechsler Adult Intelligence Scale (WAIS) or its childhood equivalent (Wechsler Intelligence Scale for Children) is still widely used. IQ scores more than two standard deviations below the mean, that is, IQ less than 70, is considered to mark impairment. In the UK, specialist services often have a criterion that they offer assistance to people with an assessed IQ of 50 or less.

Although social functioning can be explored systematically using standardised tools, none of these is completely satisfactory. Whether these are criterion-referenced or normative, there is a degree of judgement involved in deciding what 'coping' means. This is affected by social and cultural expectations, including the tolerance of the social environment to unusual behaviour.

The British Psychological Society has criteria for impairment of social functioning based on whether the individual requires significant assistance to provide for their own survival (eat, drink, keep clean, warm and clothed) and with their social adaptation, including problem solving and social reasoning (Professional Affairs Board of the British Psychological Society 2000).

Challenging Behaviour

This is recurrent behaviour that is problematic because it is physically dangerous and it interferes with learning and opportunities to access normal activities. It includes aggression, destructiveness and self-injury. It arises in 10–15 per cent of people with 'learning disability' and the incidence peaks in young adulthood. Challenging behaviour makes it more difficult to assess and deal with other problems. Containing challenging behaviour demands a great deal of effort and financial resource.

Challenging behaviour can result from pain and discomfort due to untreated medical conditions. It is important to know this. Full assessment of challenging behaviour, especially in people with marked impairment in the ability to communicate, is a specialist skill involving functional behaviour assessment. There are a number of tools that can be used to assist, but it is always based upon precise description of the behaviour, the environmental context in which it arises, and the responses that are made to the behaviour.

Autism Spectrum Disorder

Autism was a neglected disorder in the past, but there have been high levels of interest in it more recently. Increased rates of identification of ASD have led to suggestions that there might be an epidemic in progress. It is almost certain that the prevalence of ASD is reasonably stable, but that diagnostic practices have changed, and that more people now come forward for help with the condition.

There are a number of traps associated with the diagnosis of ASD. ASD is a risk factor for a range of other conditions such as eating disorders, OCD and psychosis. ASD is protean, and it is tempting to attribute all psychiatric symptoms present to underlying ASD. In fact, symptoms of other disorders should be assessed and treated in their own right. On the other hand, the possibility of ASD is sometimes dismissed if there is major trauma in the background, such as childhood sexual abuse and/or significant neglect. Abuse is just as important for someone with ASD as it is for anybody else, but it is highly unlikely to account for stable ASD features. Therapeutic responses to abuse may need adjustment if the person has ASD.

All studies show a higher prevalence of ASD amongst males than females, but the extent of the difference varies widely. There is general agreement that ASD tends to manifest somewhat differently in women. They appear to be better at imitation of social behaviour than men with ASD, and they are more likely to have a special friend. Intense and narrow interests are equally common in both genders, but women are less likely to have preoccupations that are unusual in nature. Women with ASD often have a rich and vivid fantasy life, which commonly involves multiple imaginary friends. Overall, the presentation of ASD in women is less dominated by social dysfunction. Furthermore, it is common experience that the threshold of severity of symptoms leading to referral of women with suspected ASD seems to be higher than for men, which suggests that there is a problem in recognising the possibility of ASD in women.

Finally, structured interviews are useful to help make the diagnosis, but they will not pick up other disorders that can occur alongside ASD. Use of a structured instrument may be necessary, but it is not in itself sufficient to make a complete assessment.

The Royal College of Psychiatrists (RCP) publishes guidance on the diagnosis and management of autism in adults (e.g. Royal College of Psychiatrists 2014). This is available free online. They suggest that during assessment interviews, probes should be made about three particular areas:

- *reciprocal social interaction* (relationships at school/work, being bullied or annoyed beyond endurance, understanding of others, and friendships);
- *communication* (language delay, unusual speech, non-verbal expression);
- *rigidity and repetitive interests* (hobbies, interests and preoccupations).

There are a number of structured assessment instruments for ASD. The most widely used are the Autism Diagnostic Interview-Revised (ADI-R) (lengthy to administer, but regarded as the international gold standard), the Autism Diagnostic Observation Scale, 2nd Edition (ADOS-2) (complementary to the ADI-R) and the Diagnostic Interview for Social and Communication Disorders (DISCO) (also lengthy to administer, but aimed at broader assessment than just ASD). None of these instruments are practical or appropriate for use by general psychiatrists (as specialised instruments generate misleading results when administered infrequently by non-specialists), although structured interviews can be used as a checklist without generating a score, to ensure that you ask a comprehensive range of questions.

There is a list of other structured instruments in the RCP document.

Attention Deficit Hyperactivity Disorder

This is the most controversial of the neurodevelopmental disorders. In part this is because treatment has sometimes involved giving abusable drugs (i.e. stimulants) to adults and children. The lack of a clear boundary to the disorder (because it is dimensional and developmental in nature) exacerbates concern about treatment and the medicalisation of life. In part, concern is due to the overlap between ADHD and other problems involving emotional dysregulation and difficult behaviour. In part, it is because for most people, the disorder improves during adolescence (although it is common for some features to persist well into adulthood). Consequently, the adult features are somewhat different to the childhood features. Hyperactivity is more prominent in children, inattentiveness in adults.

Problems due to ADHD are usually evident at school, even if no diagnosis is made. Problems peak at about ten years of age, and then improve in the teenage years. Adult-onset problems should be assessed with caution and with a low threshold of suspicion of a different diagnosis altogether.

The most common source of diagnostic confusion is the overlap between ADHD in adults and emotionally unstable personality disorder, impulsive type (borderline personality disorder). Whilst ADHD is usually most troublesome before puberty, symptoms due to borderline personality disorder tend to be at their worst in the late teens and early twenties. Although ADHD in adults can cause problems in relationships, this is due to the impact of the core features of hyperactivity and inattentiveness. In borderline personality disorder, the core problem is in relationships with others. Things are complicated by the fact that the disorders can occur together (notwithstanding DSM-5 caveats set out below).

Although people who are convinced that they have ADHD and that their future happiness depends on being prescribed stimulants are prone to strike a rhetorical position in an assessment interview (see Chapter 16), other patients and families minimise symptoms such as an inability to concentrate, and problematic behaviour in class or at work, because of shame and the implication of a lack of self-discipline (or poor parenting).

In line with first principles, it is important to seek hard information about expulsions and sackings, specific examples of hyperactivity, patterns of behaviour on arriving home each day from school or work, and teachers' observations at parents' evenings. Context and

---

BOX 17.2 Some Features of ADHD in Adults

- Lack of attention to detail, carelessness
- Inability to focus, commencing new tasks prior to finishing old ones
- Inability to organise activity or to prioritise
- Recurrently mislaying objects
- Forgetfulness
- Restlessness and edginess
- Excessive talkativeness, speaking out of turn, recurrently interrupting others
- Labile mood and irritability
- Intolerance of stress
- Impatience
- Physical risk-taking, for example, consistently driving too fast

---

the patient's reactions to their symptoms are important. Walking around in class inappropriately occurs in ADHD and conduct disorder. Obeying a teacher's instruction to sit down, only to get up again shortly thereafter, is compatible with ADHD. Swearing at the teacher suggests oppositional-defiant disorder. Embarrassment at inattentive and hyperactive behaviour is the usual reaction in ADHD. Basking in peer approbation for defiance is suggestive of conduct disorder.

Some of the features of ADHD in adults are set out in Box 17.2

There are no generally recommended diagnostic instruments for ADHD in adults. There are a number of screening instruments, such as the Adult ADHD Self-Report Scale-V1.1 Symptoms Checklist from the WHO Composite International Diagnostic Interview (ASRS-V1.1) (WHO 2003), but these are strictly an adjunct to careful assessment and clinical judgement. In order to make a diagnosis of ADHD, the symptoms must be evident in a range of settings, causing problems in social, educational or occupational performance. According to DSM-5, autism and ADHD can occur alongside each other. However, DSM-5 specifically excludes ADHD if symptoms arise *de novo* during psychosis or if they are better explained by a different co-occurring disorder, particularly personality disorder.

The biggest problem for clinicians in making the diagnosis of ADHD in adults is that the symptoms are non-specific, and many of them arise in a range of other disorders. One of the many criticisms of DSM-5 when it was published was the loosening of diagnostic criteria for ADHD. Some felt that this increased the risk of misdiagnosis, particularly the risk of mistaking a mood disorder for ADHD.

The other key problem is that some authorities believe that, in those individuals where it is difficult to get a clear developmental history, the only way of confirming the diagnosis is a trial of treatment. The problem with this is that low to moderate doses of stimulants make most people feel better than they did before. There is an old adage in general medicine that you cannot proceed from treatment to diagnosis, and this illustrates why. Co-incidence and non-specific treatment effects mean that diagnoses made this way are more likely to be wrong than right.

In our opinion, it is not sufficient to confirm a developmental history of ADHD symptoms. It is also important to be sure that there is not another disorder present that provides a better explanation for the symptoms and therefore a more appropriate treatment.

Tourette's Syndrome

Tourette's syndrome is the severest form of tic disorder. It is named after Georges Gilles de la Tourette, a student of Charcot who was the first to identify the condition. He called it 'la maladie des tics'. It is often regarded as the most 'neurological' of the neurodevelopmental disorders seen by psychiatrists, because the primary features involve the motor system. The symptoms have significant overlap with other neurological and psychiatric disorders.

Tics are sudden, rapid, recurrent, non-rhythmic motor movements or vocalisations involving a group of muscles. They are preceded by a premonitory urge that can be resisted for short periods, although this causes rising discomfort. The person is aware of the tics, and may be embarrassed by them. They are conventionally classified into simple motor tics (such as blinking, shrugging or grimacing), complex tics (such as hand gestures or twirling around) and vocalisations or phonic tics. The latter may be simple (grunting, sniffing or throat clearing) or complex (words or phrases, including echolalia and coprolalia). Echolalia is the repetition of elements of other people's speech; coprolalia involves use of socially inappropriate language such as swearing. These speech features are present in less than 15 per cent of people with the diagnosis. Box 17.3 sets out the differences between tics, stereotypies and mannerisms.

Tics are common in childhood, affecting about 10 per cent of pre-pubertal children. The age of onset is between four and ten years. Tics vary in frequency, severity and manifestation over time (including day to day), and they often fade during adolescence and early adulthood.

Tourette's syndrome involves multiple tics. To make the diagnosis in adults, the onset should be in childhood, and there should be both motor tics and vocalisations (although they need not be present simultaneously). Tics should occur on most days, and usually are evident daily. Males are much more likely to be diagnosed with Tourette's syndrome than women. About 1 per cent of the population in Western countries have Tourette's syndrome to some degree, and about 1 in 1,500 people have the most severe form. Symptoms may

---

BOX 17.3 Stereotypies and Mannerisms

Stereotypies differ from tics in that:

- There is no premonitory urge.
- They are not resisted and may be pleasurable.
- The movements may be prolonged.
- They are rhythmic.
- They tend to be fixed and stable over time.
- They are complex and may involve multiple muscle groups.
- They may have a neurological cause.
- Examples include hand flapping and head banging.

Mannerisms differ from stereotypies in that:

- They are unusual ways of executing complex purposeful behaviours.
- They are an idiosyncratic way of carrying out normal activity.
- They do not have a neurological or other physical cause.
- Examples include unusual walking gait and idiosyncratic accents of speech (distinct from dysarthria/regional or national accent/isolated mispronunciation of words).

improve with age, but they are often chronic. In 10 per cent of those affected, the disorder is progressive.

With regard to the way that the condition progresses with time, simple tics precede complex tics, and motor tics precede vocalisations. Early tics tend to start with the head and neck and spread distally. Tics are worsened by stress. They do not necessarily disappear during sleep.

Obsessive-compulsive and ADHD symptoms are common in people with Tourette's syndrome and their relatives. First-degree relatives are said to have an increased risk of ASD. Tourette's syndrome tends to run in families.

In assessing Tourette's syndrome, it is important to get a clear history of the movements, specifically:

> *How did they start, and at what age?*
> *Site and progression of movements*
> *Changes in frequency and form over time*
> *Factors that improve or worsen movements*
> *Is there a premonitory urge and/or resistance?*
> *Do they cause distress? Are activities avoided because of them?*
> *Are there physical consequences?*

On first diagnosis, a neurological examination is necessary. If there are movements or neurological findings other than tics, the opinion of a neurologist is needed. It is well recognised that Tourette's syndrome can present for the first time in adulthood, even in middle life. Particular care is needed to exclude other psychiatric or neurological diagnoses under these circumstances. In our experience, people who are referred as adults with an apparently recent onset of Tourette's syndrome invariably turn out to have had motor tics from childhood. Tics can be suppressed for periods of time. They may not be recognised as tics by others. People often find a way of making a tic seem less unusual, which is why the condition can pass undiagnosed until adulthood. What has usually changed is the emergence of a vocal tic, particularly coprolalia.

Giving the Diagnosis

It is possible for general psychiatrists to make neurodevelopmental diagnoses, but there is a need for a high degree of certainty, as these are not conditions that are likely to resolve after intervention. There are significant long-term implications. Patients and their families may have to make irrevocable decisions on the basis of your assessment. Naturally enough, they are likely to be keen to get a diagnosis and a plan for the future. Nonetheless, it is important to say that you do not know until you definitely do. It is tempting to talk through your own provisional conclusions with the patient and/or family. This is unhelpful until you have decided that the person definitely has the disorder. People will weigh any factors you mention for themselves, and they are likely to make their own judgement. This may pre-empt a different conclusion at a later stage, leading to the difficult task of unmaking a diagnosis.

A diagnosis of a neurodevelopmental disorder is not always a surprise or bad news, but sometimes it is. Medical students are often taught to give bad news slowly, moving from the anodyne through to the actual message via a series of incrementally alarming statements. In our experience, this is not the best way to do it. The advice is a reaction to medical brutalism: a friend of ours, a doctor, was informed that he had unexpected late liver metastasises by a radiologist who said during an ultrasound examination 'Well, the good news is it isn't gall stones ...' Obviously, that was not the way to do it either.

Generally speaking, it is as well to get to the point quite quickly, and then to give the patient and family plenty of time to think about what they have been told. They should have the opportunity to ask questions. It is good to give them information to read, which these days means information on websites. They usually value the opportunity to come back and ask more questions. One question that arises very regularly is whether the condition is genetic. It is as well to anticipate this line of questioning because the answer is complex, and the implications (or lack of them) for other family members may be difficult to explain.

Main Points in This Chapter

1. Non-specialist psychiatrists can carry out neurodevelopmental assessments and make relevant diagnoses, but care is needed to avoid misdiagnosis.
2. Neurodevelopmental diagnosis is dimensional, not categorical.
3. There is significant overlap between these disorders, and psychiatric co-morbidity is common.
4. Neurodevelopmental diagnoses should not be made where there is another diagnosis that more comprehensively accounts for the overall picture.
5. Neurodevelopmental assessment is based on the principles set out elsewhere in this book, with extra items related to the particular nature of the disorders.

Chapter 18

Personality

Personality is an intuitively simple construct that is well understood by most people, so it is perhaps surprising that theoretical and practical issues concerning personality are amongst the most difficult in psychiatry. Personality is important. It is impossible to practice psychiatry satisfactorily without a good understanding of personality. Empathic understanding of others depends upon an appreciation of the different types of personalities, and of the range of ways in which people experience the world as a consequence. No one can make a credible diagnosis of personality disorder unless they understand normal personality.

Personality is more than just the backdrop against which mental disorder plays. Personality profoundly shapes symptoms and behaviour. It creates those personal vulnerabilities that contribute to mental disorder and the personal strengths that help people to find a way back to good health.

Understanding the patient's main personality characteristics is an essential part of every psychiatric assessment. This is made difficult by three problems:

- Psychiatry has no generally accepted model of personality. There is a theoretical muddle. Consequently outsiders often find psychiatrists' attitudes to personality problems hard to understand.
- Very few people can accurately describe themselves as they are experienced by others. The assessment of personality, therefore, depends on a degree of inference and, in cases where personality issues are significant, access to more than one account. Simply relying on the patient's own account is seldom sufficient.
- Some personality disorder diagnoses have a pejorative implication that has survived the repeated application of less stigmatising euphemisms. The whole diagnostic group can be misused to pass a value judgement upon a patient or to diagnose unpopular patients out of mental health services. Whilst it is difficult to abandon the concept of personality disorder completely, the tendency for 'personality disorder' to imply 'unworthy' creates obstacles to objectivity and to acceptability for patients.

Models of Personality and Personality Disorder

Personality is that range of characteristic behavioural responses that a person deploys to cope with the world and their feelings. The greater the range and variety of responses within this behavioural repertoire, the more likely it is that the person will be able to respond adaptively to novel situations and to stresses. People with personality disorder have a limitation in their behavioural repertoire, so that their responses in some (or most) situations are maladaptive.

The various ways of thinking about personality and personality disorder can be broadly divided into three types of models: trait, categorical and structural. They are not necessarily mutually exclusive, and there are strengths and weaknesses in each.

Trait Models

In these models, behavioural characteristics are seen to group together as traits, each of which exists on a continuous spectrum. An example would be the tendency to show anxious responses. Some people only react anxiously under serious threat, whilst others show it on minimal provocation. The majority of people are distributed on an axis between these extremes. An individual's personality is the consequence of the combination of different traits displayed to different degrees. Normal personalities are those where each trait is present near the population mean. Abnormal personalities have one or more traits at the extreme.

Personality traits can be measured reliably using standardised instruments. There is a plausible link with behavioural genetics. It is possible to breed aggressive dogs or anxious mice, and family studies in humans suggest that behavioural traits are at least partly inherited.

There are some weaknesses with this type of model. It is unclear whether personality traits exist as independent behavioural variables or whether they are artefacts of psychometric tests. Traits can be broken down into smaller, more numerous components or brought together to construct fewer, larger variables. Individuals with similar psychometric personality profiles can be quite different, suggesting that these models are missing something. Personality develops and changes throughout life, but trait models can only describe this; they cannot easily incorporate developmental factors.

Categorical Models

These suggest that personality characteristics cluster together, creating distinctive types, and specific personality disorders, for example the tense, anxiety intolerant, socially insecure avoidant personality that is included amongst the personality disorders in both ICD-10 and DSM-5. The approach has face validity. For example, one regularly encounters people with typical obsessional personalities or narcissistic personalities. Personality typologies generate operational criteria. They are useful in research and in operationalising personality disorder diagnoses, and this is the approach used in ICD-10 and DSM-5.

The problem with categorical models of personality is that they fail to describe the full diversity of human personality and personality disorders. When diagnostic criteria are applied to populations of patients, some people meet criteria for more than one specific personality disorder, whilst others meet the general criteria for personality disorder, without meeting the criteria for any specific category. Some categorical personality disorder diagnoses, such as 'psychopathic personality' are incredibly stigmatising; no anti-stigma campaign could plausibly encourage the public to employ or marry someone with this diagnosis. No one appears to believe that categorical models are satisfactory, and yet they persist as the dominant way of thinking about personality difficulties within psychiatry.

Structural Models

These models rest on the hypothetical existence of underlying personality structures that determine behavioural responses. Both psychoanalysis and CBT use implicit structural models.

According to psychoanalysis, personality mainly consists of unconscious structures and mechanisms generated by childhood experience through, for example, the resolution of unconscious conflicts and the formation of internal parental objects. CBT, on the other hand, rests on the belief that behaviour is determined by learned cognitive attitudes to oneself and the world, which lead to rapid automatic thoughts beyond awareness.

Both of these traditions have produced concepts of enduring importance in understanding personality development. They share a weakness in that it is difficult to verify that their implicit structures actually exist. CBT enjoys greater credibility than psychoanalysis, as the efficacy of the associated treatment is more readily demonstrable.

Personality Disorder in DSM-5 and ICD-10

During the development of DSM-5 (American Psychiatric Association 2013), there were significant disagreements over the most appropriate approach to the classification of personality disorder. Eventually, there was no change to the approach used in DSM-IV, though it was acknowledged that it was unsatisfactory. The published definition is:

> Personality disorders are associated with ways of thinking and feeling about oneself and others that significantly and adversely affect how an individual functions in many aspects of life. They fall within 10 distinct types . . .

The current version of the ICD-10 (World Health Organization 2016) definition of personality disorder is a more detailed, and slightly wider, version of the same approach:

> includes a variety of conditions and behaviour patterns of clinical significance which tend to be persistent and appear to be the expression of the individual's characteristic lifestyle and mode of relating to himself or herself and others. Some of these conditions and patterns of behaviour emerge early in the course of individual development, as a result of both constitutional factors and social experience, while others are acquired later in life. Specific personality disorders . . . mixed and other personality disorders . . . and enduring personality changes . . . are deeply ingrained and enduring behaviour patterns, manifesting as inflexible responses to a broad range of personal and social situations. They represent extreme or significant deviations from the way in which the average individual in a given culture perceives, thinks, feels and, particularly, relates to others. Such behaviour patterns tend to be stable and to encompass multiple domains of behaviour and psychological functioning. They are frequently, but not always, associated with various degrees of subjective distress and problems of social performance.

It is obvious that 'significantly and adversely' and 'extreme or significant' involve value judgements by the assessing clinician. It follows that the difference between normal and disordered personality is not clear-cut, and that there is a borderland between the two. Personality disorder may only become manifest when the environment makes demands that the person cannot meet. For example, some impulsive aggressive young men, with a need for external structure and controls, function well in the army, but fall into a chaotic, aimless and delinquent lifestyle on returning to civilian life.

In the process of developing DSM-5, the task force almost adopted a completely different model of personality and personality disorder, known as the Five Factor or CANOE model. In the end, it was rejected, but it is set out in the DSM-5 section for research entitled 'Emerging Measures and Models'. It is a trait model that identifies 30 traits, grouped together into five major clusters of six traits each. The five groups match the acronym:

> **BOX 18.1** The 30 Elements of the Five Factor (CANOE) Model
>
> Conscientiousness: *Competence; Order; Dutifulness; Achievement-striving; Self-discipline; Deliberation*
> Agreeableness: *Trust; Straightforwardness; Altruism; Compliance; Modesty; Tendermindedness*
> Neuroticism: *Anxiety; Hostility; Depression; Self-consciousness; Impulsiveness; Vulnerability to stress*
> Openness to experience: *Fantasy; Aesthetics; Feelings; Actions; Ideas; Values*
> Extraversion: *Warmth; Gregariousness; Assertiveness; Activity; Excitement seeking; Positive emotion*

Conscientiousness
Agreeableness
Neuroticism
Openness to experience
Extraversion

There are no categories in the model, which is intrinsically dimensional in nature. Personality disorders are considered extreme variants of these traits, none of which is intrinsically abnormal. Box 18.1 sets out the six elements of each of the clusters. The mathematical symmetry of the model suggests that the elements do not necessarily correspond to mutually exclusive and collectively exhaustive human characteristics.

Assessing Personality

In the light of the competing models, the lack of pathognomic features, and the use of normative concepts, it is understandable that, from the psychiatric point of view, the whole area of personality is ambiguous and difficult. It is clear that the potential for making errors in assessing personality is considerable. There is a particular risk of deciding that anyone who is unpleasant, or who is disliked by the psychiatrist, has a personality disorder, that they are beyond psychiatric assistance and that they can be excluded from treatment. This strategy is seductive but inappropriate because it solves problems for psychiatrists but creates them for patients.

Box 18.2 sets out a few factors that are helpful to bear in mind when thinking about personality development. They are uncontentious and do not rest on any particular theoretical assumptions. We have found them useful clinically in linking current problems with historical factors that might have caused them.

Given that most people are not able to give a clear account of their own personality, assessing personality is based on four sources of information:

- The recognition of patterns of behaviour from the history.
- Collateral information (from friends or family).
- Records (school reports, social services records, GP records, etc.).
- The interaction between patient and psychiatrist.

Naturally, it is not necessary or desirable to access all these sources of information for every patient. According to how important or difficult the personality issues are, in attempting to clarify the nature of the problem, the assessing psychiatrist moves progressively down this list.

BOX 18.2 Some Factors to Bear in Mind about Personality Development

- A neonate is not a blank sheet. People are born displaying broad temperamental characteristics, which are stable in childhood and beyond. Personality is partly constitutional. However, the existence of these persistent characteristics does not imply that personality is fixed from birth. They are modified by both positive and negative environmental influences.
- These temperamental characteristics affect parental behaviour. A parent handles each of their children differently. The child is not a passive recipient of parenting. Child and parent shape each other's behaviour.
- Personality develops through the child's responses to a series of developmental challenges. These arise biologically (because people grow and age, and capabilities change over time) and environmentally (because people encounter new situations which demand behaviours outside of their repertoire). Early in life these tend to be simple but profound challenges, and they become progressively more demanding and complex over time. Developmental challenges come thick and fast in the early years and more slowly with age. They continue throughout life into old age.
- These challenges proceed in a stepwise fashion and they are repetitive.
- Some developmental challenges, such as childhood abuse experiences, can derail some aspects of personality development, although this is not inevitable. The degree to which adverse experiences lead to permanent personality problems is probably contingent on a host of positive and negative contextual factors.
- These processes create new behavioural responses and shape the available behavioural repertoire of personality. The range of new behaviours depends upon constitutional, family and social factors. Not all children are capable of developing all possible behaviours. The resolution of later challenge has a relationship with the response to earlier challenges. Consequently, some types of problem can get worse over the years.

The recognition of patterns of behaviour as the history unfolds is straightforward, if you know what you are looking for. For example, hints that the person is an anxious perfectionist suggest that they might have some marked obsessional traits. This becomes a hypothesis, and you look for evidence of attachment to routines, dislike of change, intolerance of ambiguity, checking behaviour and so on. If this is not volunteered, it is reasonable to probe:

'Do you like a well-ordered routine?'
'Do you dislike untidiness?'
'Is it difficult to finish things unless they are just right?'
'Do you like to check things?'
'Does this annoy other people?'

These are leading questions, and you have to be careful not to lead the patient into a false positive response. Some degree of obsessionality is extremely common in the general population and it is certainly not intrinsically pathological. However, the technique will often expose behaviour and personality characteristics which would not have been volunteered, either because their relevance is not obvious (why would anyone think that a lifelong habit of avoiding stepping on the cracks between paving stones was relevant to anorexia nervosa?) or because of embarrassment (how many adults will spontaneously disclose to a stranger that they still avoid stepping on cracks between paving stones?).

Any hypothesis must be open to refutation as well as confirmation. If the other features are not present then the hypothesis must fall. Even if all features *are* present, there must be evidence that they are lifelong and continuous, or at least that they repeatedly arise under similar circumstances.

It is the experience of interviewing a lot of people that teaches you most about personality and the range of characteristics that tend to cluster together. A lot of people with obsessional traits have to make sure that their shoes are kept in neat rows, carefully lined up with each other. This kind of information is not in the textbooks but it can be learnt from talking to patients. However, in the first instance, the best source of information about characteristics that tend to cluster is the personality typologies in ICD-10 and DSM-5.

People who routinely behave badly towards other people tend not to say so. They tend to rationalise their own behaviour and blame everyone else. Whilst this is one reason for talking to family and friends, it is not the main reason. People who are exploitative or aggressive or otherwise pathologically self-centred usually expose this by the way that they talk about themselves (usually as implausibly unfortunate life-long victims) and about others (who are reported to be uniformly unreliable and uncaring). The point about informants is that they have a clearer understanding of the person's habitual interpersonal behaviour than the patient themselves. The psychiatrist will invariably have formed a hypothesis about the patient's personality from the initial interview, and talking to informants allows this to be tested and/ or refined. However, in the area of personality, informants are particularly likely to come with an axe to grind, for example to emphasise their opinion that the person is ill and that the behaviour is not their fault, or to offer a causal theory ('His mother had a terrible shock when she was pregnant'). It is especially important here to hear about what the patient actually does: specific behaviour rather than interpretations of the origin or purpose of this behaviour.

It has become increasingly difficult to access old records in recent years. Of course, you need the patient's permission to do so, but many records seem to have been destroyed. Some institutions, such as certain types of schools, have become very nervous over allegations of child abuse in the distant past, or over failure to take action over evidence of child abuse. This means that precisely the kind of records that you most want to see are the most difficult to obtain. Nonetheless, it is still worth the effort. Contemporaneous accounts are invaluable and can provide a wealth of information. Some people keep their old school reports, and they are always worth looking at.

The final source of information is the effect that the patient has on the interviewer. Whilst this can be a direct reflection of the way that the person interacts, it can also be seriously misleading. The trouble is that there are two personalities in the room. If a patient rapidly irritates you, this may say something about their interactions or it may mean you are in a bad mood. As a consequence, the whole approach demands a high level of self-awareness on the part of the psychiatrist as to the types of patients that they tend to like or dislike, and an appreciation of the impact that their own personality has on patients.

Certainly, before you conclude that some reaction in yourself is a consequence of the patient's personality, it is important to check whether they have the same effect on other people. Projection of personal failings onto a third party was a particular habit of old-style psychoanalysts. As a trainee, a long time ago, one of us was very irritated by a consultant psychotherapist who recurrently fell asleep during supervision. On being woken, he would explore what it was about the trainee that had made him fall asleep. Broader attitudes and preferences of clinicians also matter. It is important to bear in mind that one doctor's charming rogue can be another doctor's vicious criminal.

BOX 18.3 A Patient with a Personality Problem

Wayne was a 25-year-old man whose wife had thrown him out of the family home. He missed her and their two small children. His wife wanted the marriage to continue, but she could no longer tolerate his jealousy and violence.

Wayne's father was a merchant seaman. He was absent from the household for long periods. Wayne, as the eldest of four siblings, was close to his mother, a woman who confided in him about her persistent depression. When his father was at home, he drank heavily. Sometimes he beat his wife. Wayne was frightened of his father, and he was distressed at the violence he witnessed. At the same time, like all children, he craved his father's approval. Wayne learned that discord in relationships was intensely threatening. His parents' relationship provided no model for conflict resolution. Consequently, he was an anxious child, but he followed the model of male behaviour provided by his father. Bravado and aggression eased his fearfulness. He was a bully at school.

Wayne had an intense but insecure dependency on his mother. He rapidly responded with aggression in any situation that he found threatening. As a teenager, he had his mother's name tattooed on his arm, which gave him a sense of her presence.

Wayne brought his insecure dependency into his relationship with his wife. Although devoted to her and the children, he easily felt that the relationship was under threat. This expressed itself as jealousy, a fear that she was insufficiently attached to him to resist sexual advances from other men. Although he knew that this was destroying the relationship, he could not prevent himself from doubting her fidelity. In the absence of an alternative strategy to cope with his feelings, he drank heavily. As he became more intoxicated and disinhibited, his restraint failed and he interrogated his wife. When she became exasperated, he took it as confirmation of his insecurities and the result was aggression and violence. Wayne's problems appeared to be linked to developmental antecedents. This created a plausible picture of his personality difficulties that could be used to understand the problem and to develop strategies to help him to contain his behaviour.

The psychiatrist assessing him was not able to obtain this history directly. When Wayne was asked about his personality, he described himself as caring but short-tempered. Asked about his family background, he described his mother as a wonderful mum. He said that he was never close to his father because he was away at sea for most of his childhood. All of this was true, but it omitted the key qualities of the family environment. The psychiatrist interviewing Wayne was aware that jealousy and aggression were likely to be related to insecure dependency, and he formed a hypothesis to this effect. Wayne's answers to simple questions were insufficient to test the hypothesis. The psychiatrist had to probe about actual family behaviour, for example about the differences in family life when his father was at sea and when his father was at home. It was necessary to interview Wayne's wife in order to establish the continuity of his behaviour patterns from childhood through adulthood.

Having decided that the patient definitely has a personality problem (whether this is a personality disorder or some aspect of their personality that is causing them difficulties), a personality diagnosis can feel rather like a full stop. One of the criticisms of a categorical approach to personality disorder is that it gives little or no indication of what might be helpful to the patient.

When trying to understand patients' personality problems, it can be helpful to think about the likely antecedents. Box 18.3 sets out the way in which history and personality difficulties can be meaningfully linked, without getting bogged down in the minutiae of competing theoretical models. In doing this, it is important to recognise that not everyone who has a difficult childhood develops a personality disorder, and sometimes people with very disturbed personalities show little evidence of troubled childhoods. The relationship between personality development and adversity is not algebraic.

Pitfalls in Assessing Personality

The misuse of the diagnosis of personality disorder as a means of justifying the discharge of a patient is one pitfall in assessment of personality. It probably operates unconsciously, or at least without being clearly formulated, so that particular caution is required when you consider the patient to have an untreatable personality problem. There are other pitfalls.

The first trap is to base the assessment of personality solely upon the patient's behaviour in a special setting. Experience of a person in a single context, no matter how lengthy, can be misleading. This is especially true during inpatient admissions. Everyone's behaviour in the role of inpatient is altered. For example, during a prolonged stay on an orthopaedic ward, you are removed from normal daily responsibilities. You are unable to make choices about daily activities and routines. You are dependent on others for basic needs. You must cope with protracted boredom. As a consequence, a range of regressed behaviour is likely to emerge, including childish pranks, vexatious disputes over trivia, bullying and so on. This gives an impression of a grossly immature personality. However, the behaviour is determined by the situation and it is not characteristic of fixed behavioural patterns elsewhere. The factors determining regressed behaviour are just as powerful on psychiatric wards, and a judgement made solely on the basis of behaviour in an inpatient setting can be expected to be inaccurate.

The second trap arises out of the complex interaction between personality characteristics and substance misuse. On the one hand, some personality disorders are associated with substance misuse. On the other hand, intoxication, especially with alcohol, can release a range of maladaptive behaviours, including aggression, impulsivity and recurrent self-harm in the absence of major personality pathology. People who are intoxicated when interviewed can appear personality disordered, especially if the intoxication is not noticed by the clinician. Intoxication with stimulants, such as amphetamine or cocaine, can make some otherwise reasonable people remarkably unpleasant. Where there is substance abuse, assessment of personality should proceed with caution.

The third trap is related to the effects of affective disorder. Both depression and mania can persist for long periods and they profoundly alter behavioural patterns. Hypomania is a term that has no fixed definition, but to us its use should be restricted to describing those states where people are elated and disinhibited without displaying florid over-activity or manic thought disorder. The condition is obvious if you have known the person in the past, as the change in their entire demeanour is dramatic, but to strangers they can simply seem feckless, attention seeking or arrogant. Mistaking hypomania for personality disorder is one of the more common diagnostic errors that we have encountered and made. Depression can also be less than obvious, and a similar mistake can be made. Both errors are less likely if an informant history is available, but this trap never entirely goes away, and it is particularly important to recognise and acknowledge that you have made the error once new information becomes available.

Some Specific Personality Disorders

There are some tricky issues associated with particular personality diagnoses. New editions of the major diagnostic systems reframe the personality disorder categories, successive euphemisms are introduced for the most pejorative labels, and diagnostic fashions change, partly in response to alterations in the conceptualisation of different categories. The move away from categories of personality disorder based on speculative theories towards more objective descriptive groupings is undoubtedly a positive development. However, there is a difference between the concepts used in everyday clinical practice and the schemata used in formal classification systems. Some concepts have proven extremely durable, and have outlived their abolition in formal terminology.

Borderline Personality

This diagnostic category has its origins in psychoanalysis, mainly in the USA. The concept of borderline personality was not generally accepted by UK psychiatrists until diagnostic usage in the two countries started to converge after the publication of DSM-III in 1980 (they have subsequently parted company again, but that is another story). Today it is the most common personality diagnosis applied to women. DSM-5 has operational criteria for borderline personality disorder. ICD-10 uses the term emotionally unstable personality disorder, which is divided into impulsive and borderline subtypes. Both systems also have a category for histrionic personality disorder. This was previously known as hysterical personality, and the diagnosis was common in the UK until borderline personality disorder came into common usage, since when it appears to have virtually disappeared. Box 18.4 sets out the ICD-10 criteria for the two diagnoses. It is obvious that there is a good deal of overlap between them.

It is concerning that these diagnoses are seldom applied to men, as they closely parallel the sexist stereotypes that misogynists apply to women in general. In fact, you do encounter males who show these personality characteristics. However, men in general tend to cope with emotional distress by drinking, taking drugs, aggression or all three. Consequently, men with these problems tend to be categorised as 'criminals', 'alcoholics', 'drug addicts' or 'psychopaths'.

Although the borderline group of diagnoses is value-laden, there is a real personality disorder syndrome within the categories. Overlapping personality disorder typologies, including narcissistic, paranoid, borderline and histrionic, turn on the theme of an inability to cope with negative emotional experience or to form and sustain close relationships. It is true that narcissistic and paranoid personality conform to some social expectations of men, with a tendency to aggressive manifestations, whereas borderline and hysterical personality conform to some social expectations of women, with a tendency to self-harming and 'manipulative' manifestations. From the point of view of severity, narcissistic and borderline are more pervasive disorders, paranoid and histrionic less severe. In clinical practice, it is necessary to understand the nature of these disorders, but to be sceptical as to whether they are separate from each other. You have to bear in mind the complicated relationships between the categories.

Psychopathic Personality

As we have mentioned, the term 'psychopath' is the most stigmatising diagnostic label available in psychiatry, with a strong implication of dangerousness and untreatability. Like

---

BOX 18.4 ICD-10 Borderline and Histrionic Personalities

Emotionally unstable personality disorder, borderline type
'A personality disorder in which there is a marked tendency to act impulsively without consideration of the consequences, together with affective instability. The ability to plan ahead may be minimal, and outbursts of intense anger may often lead to violence or "behavioural explosions"; these are easily precipitated when impulsive acts are criticised or thwarted by others. [There is a] general theme of impulsiveness and lack of self-control. [In the *borderline* subtype] the patient's own self-image, aims and internal preferences (including sexual) are often unclear or disturbed. There are usually chronic feelings of emptiness. A liability to become involved in intense and unstable relationships may cause repeated emotional crises and may be associated with excessive efforts to avoid abandonment and a series of suicidal threats or acts of self-harm (although these may occur without obvious precipitants).'

Histrionic personality disorder
Characterised by

- self-dramatisation, theatricality, exaggerated expression of emotions;
- suggestibility, easily influenced by others or circumstances;
- shallow and labile affectivity;
- continual seeking for excitement, appreciation by others, and activities in which the patient is the centre of attention;
- inappropriate seductiveness in appearance or behaviour;
- over-concern with physical attractiveness;
- associated features may include egocentricity, self-indulgence, continuous longing for appreciation, feelings that are easily hurt, persistent manipulative behaviour to achieve own needs.

---

other terms that carry a pejorative connotation, it has proven remarkably resilient in the face of efforts to replace it with euphemisms, and proposals of new ways to understand people who are unusually anti-social. Women are less likely to be given this diagnosis than men. There is a continuing debate as to whether, within a larger group of persistently anti-social people, there is a separate psychopathy syndrome.

The current DSM-5 and ICD-10 criteria for anti-social and dissocial personality disorder are similar to each other (see Box 18.5). They are painted with a broad brush and embrace a range of types of anti-social people. Almost all unlikeable and violent men meet these criteria. The modern concept of a more narrowly defined psychopathic syndrome has its origins in the work of the late Hervey Cleckley, an American psychiatrist who identified features of psychopathy that were turned into the core items of Hare's Psychopathy Checklist (Hare 1991). Cleckley remains a controversial figure. He was also responsible for the popularisation of the concept of multiple personality disorder (now understood by some psychiatrists as dissociative identity disorder). His theoretical ideas about psychopathy were highly speculative, but his book *The Mask of Sanity* (Cleckley 1988) is beautifully written. It remains the best available descriptive account of the behaviour of 'psychopaths'. Box 18.6 sets out his definition of psychopathy.

The Psychopathy Checklist (PCL-R) has renewed interest and disagreements about a core psychopathy syndrome. Hare turned Cleckley's 16 characteristics (which relate to interpersonal, affective, cognitive and behavioural manifestations) into a 20-item

BOX 18.5 DSM-5 and ICD-10 Features of Anti-Social/Dissocial Personality Disorder

DSM-5

- Failure to obey laws and norms by engaging in behaviour which results in criminal arrest, or would warrant criminal arrest
- Lying, deception and manipulation, for profit or self-amusement
- Impulsive behaviour
- Irritability and aggression, manifested as frequently assaults others, or engages in fighting
- Blatantly disregards safety of self and others
- A pattern of irresponsibility
- Lack of remorse for actions

ICD-10

- Callous unconcern for the feelings of others
- Gross and persistent attitude of irresponsibility and disregard for social norms, rules and obligations
- Incapacity to maintain enduring relationships, though having no difficulty in establishing them
- Very low tolerance to frustration and a low threshold for discharge of aggression, including violence
- Incapacity to experience guilt and to profit from experience, particularly punishment
- Marked proneness to blame others, or to offer plausible rationalisations, for the behaviour that has brought the patient into conflict with society
- There may also be persistent irritability as an associated feature

BOX 18.6 Cleckley's Characteristic Features of Psychopathy

- Superficial charm and good 'intelligence'
- Absence of delusions and other signs of irrational thinking
- Absence of nervousness or psychoneurotic manifestations
- Unreliability
- Untruthfulness and insincerity
- Lack of remorse or shame
- Inadequately motivated anti-social behaviour
- Poor judgement and failure to learn by experience
- Pathological egocentricity and incapacity for love
- General poverty in major affective reactions
- Specific loss of insight
- Unresponsiveness in general interpersonal relations
- Fantastic and uninviting behaviour when drunk and sometimes even when not drunk
- Suicide rarely carried out
- Sex life impersonal, trivial and poorly integrated
- Failure to follow any life plan

construct rating scale. It requires a semi-structured interview, access to case notes and collateral information. There are specific scoring criteria, which are used to assess inferred personality traits and behaviours. Its assumptions are normative and based on 'traditional conceptions of personality'. The scale yields dimensional scores. The items are grouped into clusters or factors. Hare states that you need specialist training to use the scale.

There are certainly conceptual ambiguities over the PCL-R. Its concept of psychopathy rests on criminality and risk, so the instrument could be regarded as a risk assessment tool rather than a diagnostic tool for a specific personality disorder. There is also a lack of clarity as to whether psychopathy is just a severe type of anti-social personality disorder or a completely distinct syndrome, as Cleckley believed. Although PCL-R is thorough and appears objective, many of the underlying qualities said to represent psychopathy are highly subjective, for example, glibness/superficial charm, need for stimulation/proneness to boredom, a parasitic lifestyle and a lack of realistic long-term goals.

Our temperamental attachment to scepticism makes us inclined to reject the Hare–Cleckley model of psychopathy, and yet we have encountered people who conform to this typology. They are very puzzling and difficult to help, and they do seem different to other people who are simply aggressive, unpleasant or frightening. We have found familiarity with Cleckley's ideas to be helpful.

Some people showing Hare–Cleckley psychopathy are chillingly callous and indifferent. The majority are not. In fact, their ability to recurrently make convincing expressions of remorse is one of their more striking features. They not only express guilt for their misdeeds, they also explain why their behaviour was inappropriate. The startling thing is their complete inability to use this knowledge to avoid repetitions of the behaviour and its unwelcome consequences. Their callousness is inferred from what they do, as it is not evident from what they say. Over time, you gain the impression that their utterances are entirely intended to provoke an immediate reaction in the listener, rather than a reflection of what they genuinely feel. You can understand why Cleckley thought that the core problem is that their feelings are completely disconnected from their thinking. Superficial charm is a common, though not invariable, feature. It sits bizarrely with their evident lack of empathy for anyone else. It is extremely difficult to understand their motivations. Much of their behaviour appears totally irrational. This contrasts with their plausible rationalisations.

Some extremely violent and nasty people have clearly developed anti-social/dissocial personality disorder as a consequence of appallingly abusive childhood experiences. In our experience, this is not necessarily true of Hare–Cleckley psychopathy. Even after extensive investigation of their early history, it can be impossible to identify convincing developmental antecedents to explain such a severe functional disorder. Needless to say, this diagnosis is important, but it can only be made with extreme care as it has far-reaching implications.

Avoidant Personality and Obsessional (Anankastic) Personality

These two personality disorders are common. They are both marked by high levels of anxiety and by marked restrictions on the person's day-to-day functioning. However, they are not associated with interpersonal unpleasantness or anti-social behaviour. The important point is that personality disorder is not synonymous with anti-social behaviour. People with these personality problems are generally only seen by psychiatrists when they develop another difficulty, leading to a symptomatic diagnosis. For this reason, the personality diagnosis is often not made. This does not matter provided their personality has been understood, as it is important in making a range of clinical decisions.

Schizoid Personality

There is considerable confusion over aloof, odd, cerebral people. In recent times, the diagnosis of schizoid personality seems to have fallen into disuse to the point where it appears to have been completely abandoned. The concept of schizotypal personality has been isolated and removed from the schizoid rubric altogether (whereby schizotypal disorder is understood as forme fruste schizophrenia, with a degree of thought disorder and abnormal affect, but no florid schizophreniform symptoms). However, the decline in the use of the diagnosis of schizoid personality appears to have paralleled the rapid increase of interest in Asperger's syndrome and ASD.

As discussed in Chapter 17, Asperger's syndrome is a mild form of autism, not meeting the full criteria for that disorder, and without a significant impairment of intelligence. Although diagnostic checklists exist, the disorder has no clear boundaries. It is assumed to have a constitutional rather than acquired cause, and to be a neurodevelopmental disorder. It would be helpful to understand if we have simply relabelled schizoid personality or whether it is a typology separate from Asperger's syndrome. Without this clarity, we stand at risk of confusion and faddishness in our understanding of people with these problems.

Main Points in This Chapter

1. Assessment of personality is a key component of all psychiatric assessments, but not all clinical situations demand a comprehensive assessment of the patient's personality.
2. It is useful to have a developmental perspective in assessing personality, whereby current problems can be linked to their historical antecedents. This can help in understanding the patient and in predicting future behaviour.
3. Assessment of personality is rarely possible from a single interview or one source of information. A personality hypothesis has to be developed and tested.
4. There is continuing conceptual confusion about personality and personality disorder, and new ways of thinking about particular clusters of behaviour continue to develop.
5. The diagnosis of personality disorder can be misused to exclude unpopular patients from treatment. Whilst some people cannot be helped, diagnosis should not be used to solve problems for the psychiatrist.
6. Not all people with personality disorder are anti-social, unpleasant or, for that matter, untreatable.

Drawing It All Together

Assessment does not just involve systematic collection of information and careful observation. There is eventually a need to bring information together and to make critical evaluations. One such evaluation involves arriving at a diagnosis. As discussed in Chapter 1, this is relatively straightforward, thanks to modern diagnostic systems, but it is an inadequate way of understanding the patient. It is only one part of a formulation.

There are two other evaluation tasks that are important in every case: the assessment of risk and the communication of your findings to others. Assessment of risk is complicated by some intrinsic ambiguities. The communication of findings can be difficult but it is often given scant attention in training. No one can be expected to learn how to do it well without properly understanding the task. The information technology revolution has made communication faster, but the attendant proliferation of proformas has inhibited the relaying of complicated and nuanced assessments accurately.

Risk and Safety

From time to time, psychiatry becomes the focus of controversy. There are accusations on themes of social control, neglect/abuse of patients, decontextualisation of human unhappiness, and lack of scientific evidence for treatments that are, it is claimed, ineffective. This has prompted the small but significant genre of psychiatric apologia, the most recent example being Tom Burns' *Our Necessary Shadow* (Burns 2013), an elegantly written book that we recommend.

At the time of writing, there is unprecedented and positive interest in mental health amongst mainstream UK politicians. It remains to be seen whether this will be sustained and whether it will prevent continued deterioration in mental health services due to consecutive reductions in funding. Despite an unusually positive public discourse about mental health, in the background there is unremitting concern amongst politicians and the media over the risk of violence and, to a lesser extent, suicide as a consequence of mental disorder.

There is no point in denying that questions of risk are difficult, including how best it should be managed. The risk of violence by people with mental illness has been wildly exaggerated, but it would be wrong to suggest that it does not exist. The risk is small, especially in comparison with the risk of suicide, but it is important. Tensions over risk have been heightened by allegations of a link between mental illness and terrorism. For some years, there has been an increasing sense amongst clinicians that they may be held accountable for events that they have little or no ability to influence. Recent developments have exacerbated this. Under these circumstances, it is hardly surprising that issues of risk and safety cause clinicians a good deal of anxiety. Modern psychiatrists live in an era of anxious practice.

In the UK, psychiatrists have access to a unique resource in the form of the National Confidential Inquiry into Suicide and Homicide by People with Mental Illness. This was first established in 1994. It collects information about every untoward death involving someone under the care of mental health services. It produces annual reports (e.g. Appleby et al. 2015), which include important trend information and recommendations to improve patient safety. Recent reports have shown a significant rise in suicide since 2008, almost certainly due to economic factors such as unemployment, and a long-term trend of a reduction in homicides by people with mental illness.

Unfortunately, evidence has little impact on policies and procedures, and some ideas that are cherished by those who control services are either questionable or simply wrong. For example, it may appear obvious that risk assessment using psychometric instruments is the key to the prevention of untoward events. In fact, it has a limited role owing to the paucity of specific and selective risk indicators and the lack of reliable risk instruments. Careful clinical judgement, together with measures to ensure well-coordinated, good quality care for all patients, are more important. Similarly, multidisciplinary discussion of risk across the largest possible range of agencies may sound like a good idea, but there are cogent arguments that group processes can take over and distort conclusions, with a diffusion of responsibility (see 'Risk Diffusion' in Chapter 15).

In recognising the limitations of risk assessment, we are not suggesting that it is unimportant or that it can be neglected. Mental health services, and the clinicians who work within them, have a duty to try to prevent bad things happening to their patients and to those around them. Whilst untoward events cannot be wholly eliminated, we acknowledge that sometimes this duty is not properly discharged by individual professionals or by whole services, and that the consequences can be catastrophic and long lasting. The point of this chapter is not to detract from risk assessment and risk management as high-priority clinical tasks, but to understand them properly in the interest of optimal safety.

Prediction

Predicting the behaviour of individual human beings is difficult. When psychiatrists try to make detailed predictions of other people's behaviour, they tend to end up looking foolish. The only halfway reliable predictor of future behaviour is past behaviour. The whole field of forensic psychiatry is based on this principle, which can be summarised as 'Careful, he might do it again'. Unfortunately, this offers little assistance when attempting to assess whether people are likely to behave in undesirable ways for the first time, which is the type of risk that psychiatrists most frequently have to worry about.

It is true that there are risk factors that are known to increase the likelihood of certain types of untoward events. For example, young males who have an alcohol problem are very much more likely to behave violently than the rest of the population. This is true of people with a mental illness diagnosis as well as the general population. The broad risk factors for violence, suicide and homicide are not changed by the presence or absence of mental illness. The large majority of people with the relevant risk factors never display untoward behaviours. Furthermore, some people who act in undesirable ways do so in the absence of any relevant risk factor. Risk factors have a limited utility in predicting individual behaviour. This is bound to be true when a much larger number of people are affected by the risk factors than will ever harm themselves or others.

In the UK, the whole question of mental illness and risk became a matter of widespread public concern following a series of events culminating in the Clunis report (Ritchie et al. 1994). This report explored the treatment of a mentally ill man who was well known to mental health services in London. He eventually killed a stranger, Jonathan Zito, at a tube station. There have been numerous subsequent reports on similar tragedies. These reports are in the public domain, and perusal of them is depressing, as they reveal repetitive themes. Few of these homicides could have been predicted. However, many of them might have been prevented if services had avoided certain key failings, namely:

- failure to collate information properly;
- failure to communicate adequately;
- failure to interview informants;
- failure to assertively follow up evasive and aggressive patients;

- making assumptions about patients (for example, Christopher Clunis, a young black man, was assumed to be a drug user and to be out of touch with his family, neither of which was true);
- re-diagnosing aggressive patients (in quite a few cases, aggressive patients who actually suffered from a treatable mental illness, such as schizophrenia, were re-diagnosed as suffering from an untreatable personality disorder or an allegedly self-inflicted drug-induced psychosis, and excluded from services);
- where risk is high, failure to develop a risk formulation (that is, a clear description of the nature of the risk, contextualised rather than quantified);
- failure to form a risk management plan or strategy.

To this can be added the uncommon but troubling situation where a patient has delusional or other intense feelings towards a named individual and expresses ideas about harming them, but the professionals involved do nothing to warn the potential victim so that they can take measures to protect themselves.

What all of this tends to suggest is that, whilst it may be difficult to predict untoward events, it may be possible to avoid them by observing the basic principles of good psychiatric practice. This includes being prepared to deal with unlikeable and difficult patients, as they are often at greatest risk.

The Nature of Risk in Psychiatry

Risk in psychiatry has a number of particular features:

- It is not a continuous quantifiable variable.
- It is much easier to say that a risk is 'high' than that it is 'low'.
- The risks faced by people with mental illness are heterogeneous.
- Reducing one type of risk sometimes increases other types of risks.
- There are risks to patients, to those around them and to the clinician (if he or she fails to prevent untoward events).
- Untoward events occur with a low frequency in each clinician's working life.
- Clinicians encounter small numbers of 'high risk' patients and large numbers of 'low risk' patients. Consequently, more untoward events occur amongst 'low risk' patients

Actuarial versus Contextual Risk

Risk in psychiatry is profoundly affected by a multitude of contextual factors. In the absence of reliable predictors, people cannot be put into high, medium and low risk categories that can be defined by actuarial probabilities. Risk is dynamic, and it changes over relatively short time scales. It rests upon the interplay between the individual's personality, the features of their illness and the situation in which they find themselves. Although there is a small group of people who can justifiably be described as dangerous (because they are likely to remain liable to do dangerous things in the long term), more commonly dangerousness is not embedded in the person, but in the total situation. For example, an aggressive young man with an alcohol problem may only become dangerous when he develops jealous delusions about a girlfriend who, by virtue of her own alcohol problem, does not take action to protect herself from his aggression.

It is very difficult to say that risk is low. The absence of positive risk factors does not indicate safety, and there are even fewer reliable protective factors than risk factors. It is psychologically more difficult to say that someone is safe. If you say that someone is at high risk and nothing happens, then in the eyes of the world (and, in all probability, yourself) you have been effective in containing risk. If you say someone is at low risk and something happens, you are just wrong. Because risk can change quickly, a fixed 'low risk' label can be just as problematic as a 'high risk' label. However, unless the majority of people are regarded as 'low risk', the term 'high risk' is completely meaningless.

Heterogeneity of Risk

In mental health services, risk tends to be thought of in terms of suicide, violence, self-neglect and vulnerability to exploitation, but this list is not exhaustive. Many different things can go wrong in life. For example, conspicuous bizarre behaviour may carry little direct risk to the patient or those around them, but it may carry a high risk of harm due to the reactions of others. If you are a stranger and persistently hang about near a school, there is a real risk of becoming a victim of serious violence, owing to public anxieties about predatory paedophiles.

Psychiatrists have traditionally focused on those risks that arise directly out of the patient's mental illness, for example the risks arising from suicidal thoughts as a consequence of depression, or homicidal ideas as a consequence of delusions. Not all risks to mentally ill people are a direct consequence of the illness itself. For example, unpleasant and violent men can develop schizophrenia, and they remain violent and unpleasant irrespective of their mental state. The extent to which mental health services should take responsibility for containing such risks is highly contentious. A pedantic separation of behaviours into those related to, and those unrelated to, mental illness is not always realistic. Many risk behaviours are mediated by the common non-specific factor of impaired judgement. It is not always appropriate to relieve mentally ill people of responsibility for their actions, but the relationship between mental state and risk can be difficult to pick apart. A lot of the time it is counterproductive to try to do so.

The Balance of Risks

Action to avoid one type of risk can increase other types of risks. Clearly, a failure to detect or to take notice of suicidal thoughts can mean that the patient comes to harm or dies. However, overreacting to fleeting and resisted suicidal ideas can lead to an excessively restrictive, custodial style of care, which itself can inflict real harm, and impede recovery. Most of the time, dealing with risk is about balancing competing concerns. This requires a careful assessment of *proportionality*. The clinician has to be prepared to take decisive action when the risk appears to be too great to tolerate, and has to retain a sense of proportion over the seriousness and likelihood of different types of risks. For example, failure to take action over concerns that a patient will act violently for fear that the therapeutic relationship may be damaged rarely represents a proportionate or appropriate weighting of differential risk.

Risk To Whom?

Most of the time, psychiatrists are concerned with risk to the patient. Sometimes, people who are mentally ill can represent a danger to those around them in a variety of ways. There are some ways of reacting to risk that shift the risk from person to person rather than actually reducing risk. Take, for example, an angry woman with acute mania recently admitted informally to a mental health unit. Patients like this can easily get into conflict with other patients, and there is then a real possibility of violence. Going for a walk with a member of staff can defuse the situation and reduce the risk of immediate assault. Patients in this frame of mind can also get into conflict with staff. Sending them for a walk on their own can reduce the sense of tension on the ward, and may help the patient to calm down; equally, it may expose the general public to a risk of aggression. In the latter instance, although the measure reduces visible risk as far as the staff are concerned, it actually moves the risk from one group of people to another. Furthermore, any risk to other people is also a risk to the patient, who has to live with the consequences. Inpatient staff are trained to deal with aggression, but the general public are not. As a result, assaults in public places often have worse consequences. Overall, the strategy may increase, not diminish, risk from the patient's point of view.

There is a more complex type of third-party risk, which is the risk to the clinician of censure. The objective evidence suggests that risk containment by mental health services has become no worse over recent decades, and it may have improved (the ambiguity mainly arises from a sharp increase in the number of people dying by their own hands whilst under the care of crisis resolution and home treatment teams). For example, whilst the UK trend of a decrease in the number of homicides by mentally ill people has been evident since the Second World War (Taylor and Gunn 1999), concern over safety has followed a general social trend in developed countries towards rising intolerance of risk in all areas of life. There is a backlash against this general trend following the reasoning that, if a risk-free life were possible (which it is not), such an existence would be bland, boring and ultimately meaningless. Whilst the question of risk in psychiatry is affected by this wider social debate, we work in environments where untoward events are closely scrutinised. Many psychiatrists fear that they could face career-ending sanctions if their patients behave in certain ways, especially if they commit suicide or homicide.

Ten years ago, there was little evidence that psychiatrists were likely to be treated harshly by employers or licensing authorities under these circumstances, provided they were conscientious in what they did. The key issue was whether decisions were made with reasonable care at the time, rather than whether they were right with the advantage of hindsight. Unfortunately, times have changed. Employers fear for their own reputations when things go wrong, and suspensions and pre-emptive referral to regulators in the absence of evidence of inadequate practice are becoming more common. The media tend not to have a sense of complexity or fair play, and the real risk of a mauling in the regional or national newspapers and/or the broadcast media generates a lot of general twitchiness amongst clinicians.

As a consequence of this background, in real life risk assessment is sometimes more concerned with protecting the professional than with making judgements in the best interests of the patient and those around them. This has a wide range of untoward effects, as making risk judgements, and deciding to tolerate an acceptable level of risk, is a necessary part of all mental health practice. We have an ethical duty to bite the bullet, and try not to put our professional interests ahead of the interests of patients.

Some patients play on clinicians' anxieties by threatening to harm themselves or other people. This is almost invariably done with the intention of persuading the psychiatrist to do something inappropriate, such as admitting the person to hospital when they are not mentally unwell or prescribing abusable drugs. On the one hand, the psychiatrist cannot give in to threats. Compliance to the person's wishes out of fear can only lead to further threats, and to unacceptable practice. On the other hand, this has to be tempered by an awareness that some people, either because of their subculture or because of illness, have a very low threshold for using threats. The conflict can reflect the fact that the doctor has made a misjudgement. There is an essential difference between allowing oneself to be manipulated and being prepared to reconsider a decision, despite unreasonable behaviour.

Low-Frequency Events

One of the problems in trying to prevent low-frequency events is that it is almost impossible to gauge how effective you are. If none of your patients are involved in untoward incidents, you do not know what would have happened if you had not intervened. If your patients *are* involved in such incidents, you do not know how many more would have been if you had done nothing.

Low-frequency events do not happen at regular but at widely spaced intervals. They tend to cluster. Think of a Geiger counter measuring background radiation; it tends to click sporadically with periods of silence. Most psychiatrists experience occasional 'epidemics' of untoward events amongst their patients. It can be hard to tell whether something has systematically gone wrong with your clinical practice, or whether this is just an artefact of low probability statistics (given that both are possible).

There are relatively few patients in the average psychiatrist's case load who are regarded as 'high risk', and conscientious teams put a good deal of effort into these patients. There are many 'low risk' patients. If we assume that the assessment of low risk is generally accurate, each individual patient is unlikely to do anything untoward, because their risk exposure is small. The clinician has a different risk exposure, as contact with a very large number of low risk patients means that some will be involved in untoward incidents. In fact, given that the average clinician is unlikely to have more than one patient commit homicide in their entire career, such events are as likely to occur amongst 'low risk' patients as amongst 'high risk' patients, if not more so.

There are two ways of misinterpreting this. The first misinterpretation is to say that risk assessment is therefore a waste of time. There is nothing about these differential probabilities that says it is impossible to minimise the chances of an untoward event amongst those at high risk. It does explain why untoward events are impossible to eliminate completely.

The second misinterpretation is to conclude that there are no 'low risk' patients and to develop a very cautious style of clinical practice. For example, as a group, patients under the care of psychiatrists are more likely to kill themselves than the rest of the general population are. You could therefore say that all of your patients are at raised risk, and this would be true. However, attempts to treat all patients as at high risk of suicide would rapidly overwhelm the service, and the lack of a focus on those truly at high risk would make risk management less effective. Such a strategy would be likely to increase, not decrease, the suicide rate amongst psychiatric patients. An overzealous, custodial and restrictive pattern of care would be likely to deter people from seeing psychiatrists, which in all probability would eventually increase the rate of suicide amongst the general population.

There is a final twist to the question of 'low risk': taking a small risk repeatedly with an individual patient can be dangerous, as the risk event is then very likely to happen. It is important to recognise the difference between the psychiatrist and the patient being repeatedly exposed to a relatively small risk. The former is inevitable but the latter is unacceptable.

Risk Assessment

'Risk assessment' is a concept of ambiguous meaning in psychiatry. Unfortunately there is no alternative but to use it, as it is the standard term. It involves a process of critically weighing objective and subjective factors at a particular point in time.

The cornerstone of risk assessment, and of all clinical practice, is access to accurate and comprehensive information. Without a proper history, it is impossible to assess risk. However, access to information can be difficult, as case notes are bulky and frequently run to multiple volumes, and modern digital records can be repetitive, far from comprehensive and very difficult to navigate. The most important part of risk assessment is collating all the relevant information.

It is possible to trawl case notes, or the history that the patient gives, for risk factors. These include evidence of previous aggression or suicidality, evidence of impulsivity and lack of self-restraint, evidence of substance misuse, evidence of social isolation and a lack of social relationships, low self-esteem and an unusually strong interest in depictions of violence. This type of risk factor is relatively non-specific and increases the risk for untoward behaviours in general. There are a handful of much more specific risk factors, which are discussed below, and which carry a relatively heavy weighting for concern.

There is another process in assessing risk, equally dependent on good quality information, but requiring a more analytical approach. Patients' life histories can be understood as a narrative, and mental illness is part of that narrative. Events do not just happen to people. We all have long-term patterns and cycles of behaviour, and life histories unfold and develop. Both episodes in people's lives and whole life histories have a trajectory, a general direction of movement. This may coincide with the person's explicit intentions, but it may be completely independent of any plans or deliberate actions they take. Spotting the trajectory of a developing situation can be critical in preventing untoward events. For example, some patients show signs of heading towards a suicide attempt without ever acknowledging such an intention. A middle-aged divorced man who is depressed after losing his job, who then gives up his social activities and gives away a much loved pet is likely to be moving towards a suicide attempt, whether he has formed an intention or not. Spotting trajectories like this is one of the reasons why histories need to be pieced together in such a way as to make sense of them from a psychological point of view.

People who are planning to do something will often say so. There is every reason to ask people about their intentions. As noted above, some patients claim to be suicidal in order to manipulate the questioner, but it is usually possible to distinguish the two situations on the basis of contextual factors. Although all doctors are taught to ask depressed people about suicidal ideas, there is a greater reluctance to discuss aggressive feelings. Conversely, many psychiatrists in training seem to learn to indiscriminately ask patients 'Do you ever feel like killing anyone?' When asked as a *non sequitur*, this invites the response 'Yes, you'. It is not difficult to ask about aggression in a stepwise fashion: questions about irritability provide a useful probe. When asking about both suicidal and aggressive feelings, it can be important not to accept blunt denials immediately. A little more probing ('Are you sure?') often reveals feelings that people are reluctant to disclose.

There is a surprising general reluctance amongst trainees to share concerns over risk with patients. In general, you can learn more about the risk if you explain your concerns to the patient. The risk does, after all, belong primarily to the patient, who therefore has a right to understand your thinking about it. Furthermore, patients are very helpful partners in devising risk containment strategies, including when the risk is of violence.

Risk Assessment Instruments

There is no evidence that risk assessment instruments are helpful in everyday clinical practice, and there is some evidence that they can be misleading. Nonetheless, there are services that insist that they should be used routinely by clinicians. Some non-clinicians are enthusiastic about instruments in general, and some clinicians strongly advocate particular instruments, which encourages the non-clinician enthusiasts in an unfortunate vicious circle.

Some risk assessment instruments do have some demonstrable predictive power. The problem with them in clinical practice is threefold. Firstly, none has sufficient specificity and selectivity to be reliable, in other words they all generate unacceptably high numbers of false positives and/or false negatives. Secondly, they create a false impression of objectivity, which can deskill clinicians, who would be better relying on careful assessment and judgement based on clinical skills. Thirdly, even the limited predictive power that they have can only be relied upon when they are used in the circumstances under which they were developed and validated. For example, the HCR-20 (Douglas et al. 2013) is an instrument that has been developed to assess the risk of violence in populations of offenders. It is widely used in forensic psychiatry services and specialist personality disorder services. National Institute for Health and Care Excellence (NICE) guidance recommends it in those settings. There is little or no evidence that it is useful in non-specialist services, and its predictive power diminishes rapidly as time passes since the last assessment. In other words, it must be re-administered regularly to be accurate. It is sometimes said that it is 'better than nothing' in community psychiatric settings, but we disagree.

Where services or individuals develop their own instruments without proper validation, their use is unsupportable. Instruments are often time consuming and tedious to complete. In busy teams there is an opportunity cost attached to using them (i.e. they prevent you from doing something more useful). The time would be better spent in face-to-face contact with the patient. Some mental health professionals like to use checklists, and we are not opposed to that, but, to reiterate, the mainstay of risk assessment is skilled clinical assessment.

Nothing we have said so far should be taken to be an argument for complacency. The National Confidential Inquiry conducted a pilot study of risk assessment prior to suicide and homicide (Rahman et al. 2013). They concluded that the overall standard of risk assessment was unsatisfactory in 36 per cent of suicides and 41 per cent of homicides. Risk formulation was one of the domains most likely to be unsatisfactory.

Risk assessment is never a completed task, but needs to be thought about constantly. It is essential to remember that risk is not an embedded characteristic of individuals; it emerges from interaction between a person and their environment. Risk, and the trajectory of a situation, can alter suddenly. In order to be able to respond appropriately, you have to be able to recognise when important changes in risk have occurred.

Some Pitfalls in Risk Assessment

The biggest pitfall in risk assessment is the gut feeling, the uneasy sense that the situation is not safe and the converse sense that the situation is safer than it might appear. Gut feelings do sometimes reflect accurate intuitions over clinical situations. Where they are reliable, it is possible to operationalise them and understand what is making you feel like that. For example, if someone makes you feel very uneasy, it may be because their eye contact and body language indicate that they are preparing to attack you. In that case, it is possible to work out what it is about them that makes you uneasy. On the other hand, it may be because they are muscular, black and male, and you have a prejudice that large black men are intrinsically dangerous. If gut feelings cannot be operationalised and broken down to their constituent parts, then they are very likely to be based on prejudices.

This applies equally to a prejudice that well brought up middle-class women do not attack doctors (they sometimes do). The patients in whom we are most likely to under-estimate risk are those who are most like ourselves and those whom we most like. It is important to try to be objective about risk, and this is best achieved by discussing cases with colleagues, or other team members. This is one of the reasons why as a matter of routine all patients should be the subject of team discussion or individual supervision.

It is important that, on a case-by-case basis, one clinician holds responsibility for assessing risk, and much of the time this will be a psychiatrist. This is because team decision-making about risk is very vulnerable to uncontrolled group dynamics. Teams can persuade themselves that people are either at much higher or much lower risk than is objectively the case. There are two processes that particularly encourage this. In most teams, team members tend to agree. Therefore, there is a psychological pressure to agree with other team members' assessments. The fact that the rest of the group agrees then reinforces the index team member's conviction of the correctness of their assessment. This tends to lead to reassuring conclusions, as the view that nothing is likely to happen is almost always correct, except when it is not. However, the situation can also develop whereby team members can convince themselves that a patient who they do not like is much more dangerous than they really are, and that some other team should be dealing with them.

Risk Factors

As stated above, there are a number of non-specific risk factors that are associated with adverse events of all types, and these are largely related to social isolation, dislocation, impulsivity and having nothing to lose. This amounts to anomie, and it is sobering to realise that Durkheim's observations (Durkheim 1951) remain relevant well over a hundred years after their original publication. There are, however, a few more specific risk factors that arise amongst general psychiatric patients (there are others of relevance to specific types of practice, for example, forensic psychiatry, but they are beyond the scope of this book).

Suicide

Suicide does not occur exclusively amongst people who are mentally ill, but risk is increased by all mental illnesses. If you are diagnosed as suffering from schizophrenia, bipolar affective disorder or anorexia nervosa, then the risk that you will eventually die by your own hand rises to between 8 per cent and 15 per cent. This is a substantial risk, but it is spread over many years, so that the risk that an individual will commit suicide in a given year is relatively low.

In some countries and cultures there are identifiable protective factors. Even if a strong religious faith or a supportive partner reduces the risk, they do not eliminate it. Hopelessness is the critical clinical factor. Patients often do not express hopelessness, but you can infer it. Evidence of sorting out of financial affairs, and of preparing the environment for one's death, is ominous. People who are depressed and paranoid are particularly likely to take their own life, especially where this is accompanied by significant anxiety. Unemployment has long been recognised as conferring an increased risk of suicide in men, and debt has emerged in recent years as a major theme associated with recent rises in the UK suicide rate.

Physical illness leading to permanent pain and disability are as important as mental illness in increasing individual suicide risk. Some people commit suicide out of anger rather than depression. It can be an act of aggression, designed to hurt specific individuals. It should not be assumed that anger is only associated with violence to others.

In assessing the risk associated with a particular act of self-harm, the degree of lethality of the act is important, but so is the patient's perception of potential lethality. If the patient believed that an overdose of propranolol was likely to be fatal because they are heart tablets, the fact that the overdose was not life-threatening is irrelevant. The patient's attitude to their survival is important. Some acts of self-harm do nothing to alter the patient's situation; some improve their situation; and some make things worse. This is relevant when the person appraises their situation in the light of their survival. If nothing has changed for the better, there is a higher risk of recurrence.

It is important to bear in mind that suicide risk is not necessarily at its highest when mental illness is at its most severe. It has long been recognised that people suffering from severe depression often take their lives during the recovery phase, and that people suffering from schizophrenia are at high risk in the first few weeks after discharge from hospital. This demonstrates that suicidality is not just related to mental state abnormalities, but also to wider contextual and emotional factors.

Serious Aggression

The diagnosis of schizophrenia increases the risk that the person will show serious aggression (Brennan et al. 2000). This is an epidemiological finding. The absolute risk is small, so that the fact of a diagnosis of schizophrenia on its own is not very relevant in assessing individual risk. If you leave aside the general risk factors for aggression (male gender, substance misuse, social dislocation, etc.), there are a handful of specific mental state abnormalities that are of relevance to serious aggression.

It is well recognised that jealous delusions are particularly likely to lead to violence. The common scenario is that the patient has been interrogating their partner for months about supposed infidelity. Eventually, exasperated, the spouse says something like 'OK, have it your own way, I have been having an affair', and the patient then becomes enraged and violent. The traditional advice to spouses who are the subject of jealous delusions is to separate, but this advice is rarely followed. All partners in this situation should be warned of the dangers of false confession, even if the apparent danger seems small.

Jealous delusions are a subtype of delusions about people in the immediate environment. Such delusions are always of concern. If you think you are being persecuted or interfered with by people around you, it only makes sense that you will eventually try to sort them out. Although the media stoke anxiety about people with psychosis attacking strangers, this is the converse of the truth. The closer your relationship with a person who has delusions about you, the greater the danger. The fact that the people concerned are normally on friendly terms or in a loving relationship is not reassuring. For example, some people deal with Capgras delusions (that someone close to them has been replaced by a double) by trying to eliminate the 'replacement' in the hope that the 'original' will return.

Command hallucinations are not necessarily acted upon, and they can be hard to distinguish from obsessional thoughts. Whenever someone receives hallucinatory instructions, it is important to explore the extent to which the person feels compelled to act on them and whether there are internal restraints against obeying.

Depressed people sometimes develop delusions that it is not just them who are doomed, but those they care about too. They sometimes believe that they have brought shame or disaster on their family, or contaminated them. This can lead to 'mercy killings', often combined with a suicide attempt. Children can be victims of such homicides, as well other vulnerable dependent people, such as elderly parents or disabled spouses.

Driving

Unless you live in the USA, the most dangerous weapon that most of us possess is a motor car. Driving when unfit is a major and common risk to patients and the general public. Taking psychotropic medication substantially increases the chances of being involved in a serious accident. All mental illnesses make driving more difficult through impaired concentration, distractions such as hallucinations, impaired judgement and increased impulsivity. Depressed patients sometimes become indifferent to their own safety and drive more recklessly as a form of fatalistic Russian roulette. This is not to say that people with mental illness necessarily should not drive, but their fitness to do so should be assessed, and if they are not fit, they need to be clearly informed of this. It is also important to remember that some people habitually drive without a licence and without owning a car. Young men in particular need to be questioned closely as to whether they drive.

Child Protection, Terrorism and 'the Duty to Disclose'

There are an increasing number of circumstances where clinicians have a duty to disclose confidential information. This can cause significant problems in therapeutic relationships. If we leave aside breaches of confidentiality that are intrinsic to the use of legal detention under mental health legislation, most of the newer responsibilities relate to a risk to a third party. Few clinicians have great misgivings about warning a specific potential victim of a risk from a particular patient where there is nothing else that the psychiatrist can do to prevent an act of serious violence. However, there are more ambiguous circumstances than this.

There is general support for the principle that the protection of children should be one of the highest priorities for society in general and for health professionals in particular. At one time there was no specific duty to report to the authorities disclosures of historical childhood sexual abuse where the abuser was, or might be, in continued contact with children. This is now a well-established feature of medical practice in the UK and elsewhere. Most health professionals accept it as appropriate. This is not to say that it is uncomplicated or problem free. Where the doctor breaches confidentiality against the patient's wishes, the therapeutic relationship is invariably damaged and frequently does not survive. Furthermore, a forced disclosure can cause huge distress and permanent changes to relationships within whole families. This is not to suggest that reporting such disclosures is the wrong thing to do, but there is a cost in terms of tangible harm. The degree of effectiveness in protecting children is unclear, and acceptance of the principle is in part a reaction to a high level of concern that health professionals in the past have done too little to prevent child abuse.

There are new expectations that health professionals in general, and psychiatrists in particular, will take a role in the prevention of terrorist atrocities. At the time of writing, there is a controversy over the UK Prevent anti-radicalisation programme, which has a statutory basis and allows little discretion to the clinician. It requires that doctors refer patients whom they believe might be vulnerable to developing a radical philosophy to a de-radicalisation programme.

Some psychiatrists are concerned about a lack of evidence that people with mental health problems are particularly vulnerable to recruitment to organised terrorism; about a lack of evidence that de-radicalisation of people with mental health problems is likely to work; and about the effect of the programme in alienating sections of the population from seeking mental health treatment. People with serious emotional difficulties sometimes carry out mass shootings, and other individual acts causing mass casualties. Critics point out that only a tiny minority of people who commit these crimes adhere to a radical ideology. It is far from clear whether 'lone wolf' terrorists are inspired by radical philosophies or adopt them because they justify actions that they are drawn to for other reasons. Psychiatrists who are worried about these new responsibilities suggest that targeting particular sections of the population as 'vulnerable to radicalisation' is discriminatory and unlikely to have much impact in preventing atrocities and that the programme may prove counterproductive.

These issues are not going to disappear in the foreseeable future. It is necessary to remember that doctors owe a greater loyalty to their ethical code than to any political regime. Doctors have to weigh up carefully the risks and benefits to individuals and to the public in breaking confidentiality. They will sometimes conclude that they are ethically bound to defy political policies or even the law. The other side of this responsibility is that they then have to face the consequences.

Safety Considerations

Mental health professionals are shouted at or threatened from time to time. This is an unfortunate but unavoidable aspect of the job. Actual assaults are relatively rare. Working in the community, the greatest risks are related to road traffic accidents or being mugged. Nonetheless, to paraphrase a point made earlier, a low risk taken repeatedly becomes a high risk. There is good reason to be cautious or indeed cowardly. This not only protects you, it also protects patients. Frightened doctors make bad decisions and patients often pay a heavy price for assaulting mental health staff (insofar as they get sent to secure facilities and are treated as dangerous by those who look after them forever after).

Although a number of points about safety have been made elsewhere, the main principles in maintaining your personal safety in hospital and in the community are worth reiterating here. They cannot always be followed. If you have to break these principles, this should be done as an exercise in calculated risk-taking rather than in a spirit of blind optimism.

- When you first assess a patient, the amount of information available may be quite limited. You should insist that referrers give as much information as possible. Amongst other things, this allows you to be as clear as you can be about risk prior to the interview. If there is cause for concern, gather information about the individual from other professionals and from GP records beforehand. If another agency is involved, and can be contacted without a breach of confidentiality, this should be done before assessment. It is especially important to gather information prior to a first visit to a patient's home. It is sometimes necessary to speak to friends and relatives prior to a home visit, although this can easily compromise confidentiality. Never go alone into someone's home for clinical purposes without speaking to someone who knows them first. The best protection against unexpected aggression is good quality information.

- Some types of patients are more likely to assault a doctor. People who are aggressive when well are likely to be aggressive when ill, as are patients who are intoxicated with alcohol or drugs. Patients whose psychosis leads them to believe that there is a threat to them in the immediate environment may deal with this through aggression. Patients with delusional ideas that specific individuals are responsible for their misfortunes are likely to react aggressively.
- Before commencing an interview, you should be reasonably certain that the patient is not carrying a weapon. Interviews with aggressive patients should not go ahead if there are objects in the room that can easily be used as weapons, for example, heavy crockery or kitchen knives.
- Ensure that you can escape unimpeded. You cannot allow the patient to have control of the space. You should position yourself between the patient and the door. In the patient's own home, ensure that you cannot be locked in.
- Make sure that assistance is available. This means that there must be an agreement between yourself and other staff on how you will raise the alarm, and that they will respond to the alarm. This is reasonably straightforward in a hospital, provided you make no assumptions. The agreement on assistance should be explicitly stated between the staff on hand and yourself before the interview.
- When working in the community, either alone or with another team member, make sure that someone knows exactly where you are, and when you are due back. They need to know exactly what to do if you do not arrive on time. The latter is particularly important, as simply knowing that you are late creates a dilemma for the other person. There must be an agreement as to the threshold for regarding this as an emergency. On the other hand, you are unlikely to allow yourself to be delayed if you know that the police will be called if you are more than half an hour late.
- Be prepared to withdraw if your fear is rising or if you cannot calm the patient. If the interview is failing, for example if the patient is becoming more threatening, a break will not make things worse, and it sometimes helps.
- In the community, try to work in pairs. In a first assessment in the community, the patient is often reassured by the presence of someone they know. In the hospital, if you do not feel safe alone with the patient, have someone else with you. Make it clear at the outset who is conducting the interview and that the other person should not intervene unless invited to do so. If you are alone and you have to say something that is likely to be provocative, break and get someone else to be with you.
- If you are seeing the patient at home, let them know that you are going to visit. It is unannounced visits that most commonly trigger aggression. From the patient's point of view, the unannounced arrival of a psychiatrist at the front door is obviously provocative. If there is a good reason to visit without warning, usually because admission to hospital under compulsion is anticipated, there is no option but to speak to a family member first, even though this compromises confidentiality.
- Travel with the means to summon help, namely a mobile phone. This only works if you take care to ensure that the battery is charged. The sight of a 'dead' mobile phone is little deterrent to the determined assailant.

- Be aware of aspects of your own behaviour that are likely to convey threat to the patient. This means retaining an awareness of the patient's point of view. An angry patient is unlikely to respond well to being told he is going to be detained. Trying to argue with him is likely to be provocative. Tense body language and the invasion of personal space are threatening. Try to adopt a relaxed posture and talk slowly. If you think the patient is being aggressive out of fear, say so. Similarly, aggressive patients are frequently unaware that they are frightening others, and it can be helpful to point this out. An appearance of not listening to what the patient is saying is very frustrating. You may not be able to relieve the patient's frustration, but it will ease if they feel that their concerns are being acknowledged.
- Do not take any responsibility for physically restraining the patient unless you have been trained to do this. Hospital nursing staff are trained to do this safely. A preparedness to grab the patient is easily read in body posture, and it does nothing to reassure the patient.
- Most psychiatric services provide staff with training in 'breakaway techniques'. Attend these courses.
- Do not carry a weapon. Even a can of pepper spray can be turned against you. Producing a weapon is more likely to provoke violence than prevent it.
- A very small number of patients bear a grudge and stalk mental health professionals. It is wise to have an ex-directory telephone number, to avoid being listed under your professional name on publicly available versions of the electoral register, and to be circumspect in revealing where you live (even in terms of the general area).

Main Points in This Chapter

1. Predicting behaviour is difficult.
2. Risk assessment depends on collating full and accurate information, on assessing the trajectory of the situation as it develops and on being aware of the major risk factors.
3. Adverse events occur amongst 'low risk' as well as 'high risk' patients.
4. Adverse events are minimised by doing the job properly and by recognising that the patients we least enjoy dealing with are at highest risk.
5. Personal cowardice is the safest policy in the course of a whole career in mental health, despite the fact that the personal risks are small.

Record Keeping and Reports

At this stage, we hope that the reader is persuaded that psychiatric assessment involves far more than history taking, mental state examination and diagnosis. It is a dynamic process that lays the foundation of a therapeutic alliance. This includes the formation of a shared understanding with the patient of the nature of the problem, set in the meaningful context of the patient's life. This shared understanding does not necessarily arise immediately, and the process of achieving it can take years. On the clinician's part, there has to be a selective and critical approach to the mass of information available. The psychiatrist has to be able to identify the most important features of the overall situation, to recognise patterns of behaviour within the history and to identify the trajectory of the patient's life history. The impact of all this effort is largely lost unless both the facts and the analysis are properly recorded and communicated.

From the fifth decade of life onwards, it is very noticeable that nothing is quite as good as it used to be. There can be little doubt that this is predominantly an effect of the ageing process, but in two particular areas it is certain that the perception is correct. You eventually reach a point where you, yourself, are nothing like as good as you used to be and neither are psychiatric records.

Paper Case Notes

Paper case notes are still with us (see Box 20.1). One day, someone in authority will realise that their quality cannot be measured by their weight. Modern case notes are packed with forms: care programme approach forms, risk assessment forms, photocopies of welfare benefit forms and so on. Whatever the advantages of the use of proformas in general, their bulk is beyond dispute. This means that most people's notes run to multiple volumes, and it is very difficult to retrieve information (one could argue that risk assessment instruments record information that was much easier to access before such forms came into use). The plethora of documents gives a false impression that everything has been recorded and that it is less important than it used to be to keep clear running clinical records. The opposite is the case.

Running notes, made as the interview proceeds, are indispensable. They may be unreadable to everyone other than the author, but this is not a reason not to make them (some doctors can touch type, and should be able to make legible contemporaneous digital notes, but hardly anyone ever does). The main tenets of good note keeping are simple. Every sheet should be dated and marked with the patient's name, in case they become detached. There should be a record of where the interview happened, and who was present, each person identified both by full name and relationship to the patient/professional role. It is surprising

BOX 20.1 Paper Records Will Always Be With Us

For more than 20 years managers of mental health services have resisted improvements to case note systems on the grounds that paper notes will shortly be replaced by comprehensive electronic record systems. Computers have become ubiquitous, and hard copies of emails, faxes and printouts of electronic contact records have added to the bulk of paper notes. Most health care providers have an electronic record system. These normally have an acronym (e.g. 'The CICO system') and they are purchased amid high hopes that they will replace paper, save time and money, be easy to use and provide access to records to authorised personnel from all corners of the globe. Of course, they do have some advantages, as they can in theory be accessed out of core hours, from any point that has a link to the organisation's Intranet. Senior staff at home can even give advice based on reading the notes on their laptops. However, electronic systems are almost invariably problematic, especially when trying to find a chronological account of what happened and why. Unlike paper, digital systems crash and suffer from viruses or hackers. IT departments do not phone to let you know that the paper notes 'are down', but this is a regular occurrence with computers. Organisational structures change regularly, and invariably when organisations merge, 'the systems don't talk to each other'.

Currently in the UK, some organisations have paperless systems, but many have a combination of electronic and paper. Those that have electronic only tend to actively discourage the use of any paper record.

Digital systems are beasts that must be fed, but the single most secure piece of advice we can offer in this book is that you should assume that your need to keep some form of paper record will never disappear.

Please do not write to our publisher to say that you have not used paper records since 1985. We are aware of such practices but consider it to be a mistake.

how quickly staff turn over and how quickly everyone forgets, for example, who 'Brian' was. There should be a clear and detailed record of what led up to the patient being seen, especially in emergency situations. The source of information and its perceived reliability should be noted. There should be examples of behaviour and symptoms of concern, as discussed in Chapter 3. There should be a clear distinction made between what has been observed directly, and what has been reported. Sensitive information should be very clearly labelled as such. If an undertaking is made not to disclose information to third parties, this should be conspicuously flagged, and it is usually best to record this on a separate sheet marked 'Not to be disclosed without permission'. Such undertakings should be made with great caution. There are many legal requirements relating to data access that may override your promise.

At the end of the note, we are in the habit of having a section for conclusions headed 'Impression'. If some part of this is not disclosed to the patient, it is important to record this (although, as a matter of principle, this should only be done if there is a very serious safety concern). If third parties are told of conclusions, this too should be noted. We follow this with a heading 'Plan'. It is good practice to have such a section in the notes for every follow-up appointment, as well as assessment interviews. This helps you to think about what you are trying to do regularly and to notice when the plan is going wrong. The 'plan' section should include an explanation as to why you have made particular decisions. It is inevitable that shortcuts are taken when making notes, but some shortcuts should definitely be avoided. For example, if you are arranging blood tests, there is no point in noting 'routine bloods requested'. Each investigation should be listed, together with the result when it arrives. Similarly, you should record each of the major statements you make and any suggestions you make to the patient. It does not instil great faith if you have to ask the patient what you said or did at the last interview. Finally, each entry should be clearly marked with your name, job title and the team you work with.

Letters

Writing good letters is a difficult skill to master. They have several purposes. They communicate what you intend to do, and why, to the patient and others (usually including the referrer). They serve as a legible and clear summary of your findings and your intentions. As they accumulate and record subsequent events, they form the chronological spine of the case record. As such, they should be processed and thought-through documents rather than a simple reiteration of the 'raw' history and mental state examination.

Many services have a computerised template for routine letters and discharge summaries. The intention is to ensure that certain essential information is communicated reliably. They do achieve this end. However, they militate against the creation of a clear narrative, which is the hallmark of a good clinical letter. Indeed, when reading these templated letters, it is often hard to understand why decisions have been made. For example, when patients are seen in an emergency department, there is often a brief letter following a template, which sets out the circumstances of an act of deliberate self-harm and requests a full assessment. Without more information, it can be very hard to tell why it was felt that the patient needed to be seen, or to assess which team member might most appropriately see them. Templated letters are certainly better than a poor letter or no letter, but we prefer something less basic.

Clinical letters should tell you why the patient has presented in this way at this time. They should tell the story and they should be easy to follow. They should not be too long: around two sides of A4 paper for an assessment letter, perhaps one side for a follow-up letter. It should be easy to comprehend why the conclusions were drawn and what the treatment plan is. If the interview has not led to a full history being gathered, it should be clear what is known, but also what still needs to be found out. The test of an adequate letter is that, if you drop dead before the next interview, it should be reasonably straightforward for your replacement to pick up the threads of the case on the basis of your letter.

Very few GPs will read an assessment letter from start to finish. If you want them to do something (such as organise investigations or prescribe a drug), it needs to be clearly stated at the end of the letter, if necessary in bold type. If there are essential tasks to be carried out, such as monitoring of blood lithium levels, it should be clear as to whether you intend to do this or whether you expect the recipient to carry it out.

No one is examined on their ability to write a good letter, and we now test clinical skills through atomised testing of isolated specific tasks. Nonetheless, anyone who can write a good assessment letter should be capable of doing well in clinical postgraduate examinations. Assessments and letter writing are one of the most important ways of preparing for these exams, because they involve the full range of clinical and analytical skills (see Box 20.2).

We have tried voice recognition systems when dictating letters. At this stage of reading the book, it will cause little surprise to learn that we think that they are more trouble than

BOX 20.2 A Clinical Assessment Letter about a Difficult and Fragmentary Interview

Dear Dr Patel,

Re: Irene Wright (d.o.b.: 18/6/68)

This patient of yours was referred to the CMHT by Maria Dutton, a volunteer at the local food bank who has known Mrs Wright and her two children since July 2016. I interviewed her with Carol Penley, CMHN and Ms Dutton, in clinic on 23/12/16.

The referral did not occur because of a clinical crisis, but because the family have no money to live on, following a punitive withdrawal of Mrs Wright's welfare benefits. This fortuitously provided an opportunity to carry out a mental health assessment of Mrs Wright. She has been referred to this service on at least three occasions since 2009, but has always declined assessment.

The interview was not 100 per cent satisfactory. There were five of us in the room (Mrs Wright brought her 14-year-old daughter, Emily, with her). I did not obtain a comprehensive history, but we did manage to establish the likely nature of the problem.

As I'm sure you are aware, Mrs Wright has a long history of odd behaviour and neglect of her house, with episodes of shouting and verbal abuse. She has always been reluctant to engage with services. In 2006, the Alcohol Dependency Service treated her for three weeks as an inpatient. It is hard to pin down the severity of her alcohol problem in the past. She admits to a lifetime maximum intake of three quarters of a bottle of wine a day, but Maria Dutton is quite certain that her consumption has been more than a bottle each day recently. I could find little evidence of physical or social sequelae of heavy drinking. She denies ever having suffered withdrawal symptoms and she has never drunk daily. She does regard alcohol as a problem that she has to keep under control. There was no evidence of alcohol intoxication or withdrawal at interview.

At interview, Mrs Wright was a little dishevelled, with adequate, but not good, self-care. Her skin was reddened. She told me that she had been washing her hands with bleach, but the appearance was more suggestive of prolonged exposure to the cold. Her mood was euthymic, and she engaged pleasantly with us. She did, however, display marked thought disorder of the schizophreniform type, at times to the point of incoherence. There were copious active psychotic symptoms. It is hard to know whether her difficulty in describing these arises from her awareness that they sound very strange. She was certainly quite guarded on some subjects, and sometimes altered her descriptions of symptoms when I tried to clarify their nature.

Despite these difficulties, we did establish that she believes that an organisation implanted a probe in her brain when she was an inpatient in 2006, and that she has subsequently been used to transmit messages about forthcoming terrorist atrocities. She believes her movements are being monitored. She suffers from continuous auditory hallucinations, and paused to listen to these at several points during the interview. She told us she has to lip-read in order to distinguish speakers' voices from hallucinatory voices. She gave me the impression that she also suffers from somatic hallucinations, passivity experiences and delusions of reference, but it was hard to be certain on the basis of this interview. Despite this uncertainty, the likely diagnosis appears clear.

With regard to her social functioning, Mrs Wright has shown a degree of indifference to markedly unsatisfactory living conditions over several years, and has lately tolerated having insufficient money to heat and light her home. Emily has been living with foster parents for the past one year. Mrs Wright's son, Graham, aged 19 years, lives with her. Her description of her daily activities is unremarkable, but I suspect that it is erroneous.

There is a great deal of background information that we need to gather, and Carol Penley is going to do this over the next few weeks. The really important thing is to engage with this lady. We are going to try and help her with her benefits, and access to sufficient food to last over the Christmas break. I don't think that her primary problem has anything to do with alcohol. She is showing unequivocal symptoms of chronic schizophrenia, with a longer-term history that is compatible with that diagnosis. I don't think that there is any great urgency in getting her to take medication. Once we have sorted out some practical problems and formed a relationship with her, it will be easier to work on improving her mental state. I will review her early in the New Year, and I will let you know what happens next.

Yours sincerely

they are worth, although the software involved is clearly improving. Audio-typing remains the predominant method of producing letters. Dictaphones are small bits of equipment that seem to have a disproportionate capacity to intimidate doctors. Consequently, doctors mumble into them very quietly and quickly, which is exactly the opposite of what secretaries like. Slow clear speech makes an enormous difference. As far as possible, you should dictate the punctuation, as this makes it clearer to the secretary what you mean. You should break up the letter with paragraphs, as these make letters easier to read. Words that are unusual should be spelled out, including unusual names. When you are not speaking, stop the tape running, as long gaps are awkward on playback. When the letter is finished, say so, and when you have finished dictating, state that the tape is finished (failing to do so regularly risks the secretary missing a letter and wiping the tape). When the letter comes back for signing, always check it and correct errors. Especially look out for errors in drug doses, and bear in mind that even the most efficient secretary occasionally misses a 'not' and inadvertently reverses the meaning of a whole letter.

Good letter writing comes with practice. Following these points will help considerably, and will make the team secretary's life easier. It is worth nurturing secretarial staff. No other profession can have such an impact in making your working life more pleasant or, if provoked, a lot more difficult.

Reports

Report writing is an intrinsic part of most psychiatrists' work. Many of these are quite straightforward, for example reports to insurance companies. Others, especially court reports, are much more complex.

The first thing to think about in writing a report is whether you have permission from the patient or not. Not all reports require the patient's consent. For example, reports to mental health tribunals considering appeals against detention do not require patient consent. Most types of reports do require such permission, however, which should normally be obtained in writing.

The next question is 'What does the agency requesting this report need to know, and how much specialist knowledge are they likely to have?' Generally speaking, you should only reveal the minimum amount of confidential information necessary, even when you have permission from the patient. This is not to say that you should ever conceal relevant information, no matter how unpalatable. However, permission is often given under a degree of duress (for example, you only get your benefits if you reveal your psychiatric history), and it is wrong needlessly to expose sensitive information.

In writing reports, psychiatric terminology has to be explained or turned into more ordinary language. There is no point in reporting something that the third party is unable to understand.

Major reports, to courts or mental health tribunals, should follow a set of well-established principles:

- No matter who has requested a report, your duty is to give as dispassionate an account and opinion as possible. In court reports, your duty is to the court. You should never get involved in a rhetorical process, nor alter your opinions to the convenience of one side or the other. If you are unable to form an opinion, or if you are unable to choose between two different ways of interpreting the situation, you should say so.

- It is conventional to refer to the subject by their full name throughout court reports. It is not necessary to follow this convention in other reports.

- The report should start with a statement as to who has requested the report, and the purpose of it. If you have been asked to comment on certain aspects of the situation, this should be stated at the outset.

- In some reports (especially where you are acting as an expert witness), it is necessary to set out your qualifications and experience. You need to find out from whoever has requested the report whether you need to include a short résumé.

- Next, there should be a description of the evidence that you have drawn upon in preparing the report. When acting as a professional witness, this is likely to be your experience of treating the patient over a specific length of time. As an expert witness, it might be a single interview specifically for the purpose of preparing the report. In the latter case, you should make clear to the patient at the outset why you are seeing them and that anything they say may appear in the report. The fact that the patient was so warned should be stated in the report.

- Any records, reports, witness statements, documents or relevant interviews with third parties that have contributed towards the formation of your opinion should be listed.

- In the body of the report, it is essential to separate facts from opinions. The main part of the report should start with a factual account of the index events (admission to hospital or alleged criminal offence, for example), usually followed by the patient's account. In court reports, the offence should be referred to as 'the present alleged offence' even where the person intends to plead guilty.

- There should then be a psychiatric history followed by the background history. This need not necessarily be set out as fully as it would be in a clinical letter. However, there needs to be sufficient information to allow the reader to understand exactly why you have reached your conclusions. This section should not include opinions, though you can report here historically what your opinion was at a particular time. For example, you can state that you admitted the patient because at that time it was your opinion that they were depressed.

- There should be a description of the patient's mental state during the interview, usually the most recent interview that has occurred. Technical terms, such as 'delusions of reference' should be explained in parentheses '(the false belief that neutral material has a specific personal message)' or should be followed by a clear example from the patient's mental state examination.

- If there are complex issues or major ambiguities, it can be helpful to have a section marked 'Discussion', setting out the variety of ways in which the situation can be interpreted, allowing clarification before you express an opinion.

- Conclusions should be so headed, listed and numbered (this makes discussion of the report much easier in formal proceedings). Each numbered paragraph should contain one aspect of your opinion, with the prelude 'In my opinion . . .'. The listed opinions should move from the general to the particular, for example from whether the patient is under disability with respect to his trial ('fit to plead'), whether they have a mental illness, whether there are further psychiatric disorders present, whether there are physical factors of note, any circumstantial factors of relevance and the relationship between the mental disorder(s) and the person's behaviour, ending with any recommendations.

- You should not express an opinion outside of your professional expertise, no matter how obvious. If an opinion is based upon your general medical knowledge rather than specific psychiatric knowledge, you should say so.
- Court reports should end with a statement that the contents are true to the best of your knowledge and belief, and that you are content for the report to be placed before the court.

An important test of your ability to write a good psychiatric court report is how often you get asked to attend court. A well-written report about less serious offences will normally avoid you having to appear, as the report will be easy to understand and there will be little that the lawyers will feel able to challenge.

Reports often attract a fee for preparation, but you are mostly, in any case, more or less obliged to write them. It is easiest if you learn how to write them early in your career, which normally means asking supervising consultants if you can write tribunal reports. It is true that the task is burdensome to begin with, but this is the only way of acquiring the necessary skills.

But the Patient Might Read It . . .

These days, patients are liable to read just about anything that a psychiatrist writes about them. This only matters if you are in the habit of being disparaging about patients in letters or if you do not discuss your conclusions or your plans with them. There are a tiny handful of situations where the latter might be justified, and none at all where the former is appropriate.

At the time of the introduction of the right to read clinic letters, there was a good deal of talk amongst psychiatrists about keeping 'double records' or changing the content of letters in some other way. In fact, most patients are not overly concerned to see letters. When they are, it sometimes indicates that something has gone wrong with the relationship with the writer or the intended recipient. Some patients are curious or like to be able to remind themselves what happened.

In any case, there is nothing wrong with people wanting to see letters and notes. In fact, it is a little surprising that doctors ever thought that it was acceptable to routinely write about people without their knowledge and in the absence of any right to know what had been written. If there are statements or conclusions in reports or letters that you are uncomfortable about the patient seeing, then it can be important to understand why this is so. In general, it is better for you to tell patients face to face what you have written, no matter how uncomfortable this might be. Truthfulness, openness and frankness are well recognised to be important in relationships in general, and they are no less important in therapeutic relationships.

Main Points in This Chapter

1. Note keeping, letters and reports are important. They are tedious tasks, but the skills can only be developed with thought and practice.

2. An awareness of the purpose of these documents is helpful.
3. Clarity of writing is improved if you bear in mind the recipient's needs, including any limitations to their knowledge of psychiatry.
4. Generally speaking, it is helpful to clearly separate fact from observation and opinion.
5. If you cannot share everything in a document with the patient, there is either something wrong in your relationship with the patient or there is a high risk of an unusual type.

Afterword

Getting Alongside Patients

Working in mental health is not a good way to become wealthy. Efforts to make a lot of money through psychiatry tend to take practitioners into ethically dubious territory. In every other respect, however, a career in mental health can be incredibly rewarding. Working as a psychiatrist can offer an extraordinarily rich experience and an unrivalled window into some of the most hidden aspects of human existence. The work can be intellectually demanding, stressful and frustrating, but it is never, ever, boring.

Two things become increasingly evident as you become more experienced. Firstly, it becomes obvious that the way that you deal with patients is at least as important as what you do by way of technical intervention. The second is that over time you encounter many people who overcome devastating mental illnesses with their dignity and self-respect intact; people who may still need the assistance of professionals from time to time, but who have learned to manage their mental illness, and in doing so, have recovered. To have helped in this process is humbling.

Psychiatry: Far from Perfect . . .

One of the things that make psychiatry so interesting is that it is full of ambiguities. Working as a psychiatrist routinely presents you with dilemmas that defy simple or formulaic resolution. Dealing with such situations demands creativity and, in the absence of a right answer, you are bound to get things wrong sometimes. Working in psychiatry teaches you that the human spirit is an awesome thing, which can survive the severest mental illness. Unfortunately you also learn that it can be crushed by other people, even when they are well intentioned. It takes courage to acknowledge that your own mistakes sometimes have this effect.

Organised psychiatry has been involved in some highly questionable activities in its short history (although in all likelihood individual doctors thought they were doing the right thing at the time). Psychiatrists were deeply involved in the eugenic projects of the first half of the twentieth century. They presided over forced sterilisation programmes in the USA in the mistaken belief that they would thus eliminate mental illness from the population (Kevles 1999). They participated in selecting people for death in the Nazi camps, sometimes in the belief that they were saving other lives (Lifton 2000). In the 1950s and 1960s, they exposed patients to treatments, such as insulin therapy and narcosis, which they knew were dangerous. Unfortunately they also turned out to be ineffective. In the Soviet

Union, as recently as the 1980s, psychiatry was misused for political purposes through construing dissent as psychopathology.

Psychiatry is not alone in having such a history. Social work, psychology and psychoanalysis all have corresponding histories that, in retrospect, are shameful and indefensible. Social values are unstable, and no doubt some aspects of modern practice will appear wrong in the near future. It is difficult for anyone to protect themselves against the risk of the retrospective condemnation of history. We should, nonetheless, try to avoid causing harm in the here and now.

Whilst the examples of the psychiatric abuse cited may seem extreme, distant and unrelated to modern psychiatric practice, psychiatry is not yet in the clear. Our capacity to do harm has not been eliminated. At the time of writing, psychiatry in the UK faces many challenges to its ability to remain within acceptable ethical boundaries. For example, in the treatment of heroin dependency, a treatment objective of abstinence has replaced harm reduction on the basis of ideology rather than evidence (grotesquely labelled as recovery in the face of a rising death rate amongst heroin users); anti-terrorist programmes are drifting towards a fundamental change in the relationship between psychiatrists and the state, despite the lack of a demonstrable link between organised terrorism and mental disorder. There are other examples. Increasingly frequently, individual psychiatrists have to confront a conflict between their ethical responsibilities and governmental expectations.

Psychiatry can have more pervasive adverse effects. We stand accused of collusion with the medicalisation of everyday life. For example, the development of the concept of PTSD has been criticised as an unhelpful extension of the disease metaphor (Summerfield 2001). We have sympathy with this critique, and, in our opinion, the problems are not hypothetical.

If distress in the face of adverse social conditions is construed as an illness, with a technical solution that can only be delivered by experts, then there is an inevitable penalty for the sufferer in terms of personal helplessness. This encourages a victim mentality, in which people are angry at having been wronged, but have to look outside of themselves and their community for reparation and 'cure'. This is not to minimise the suffering of, for example, those who have been traumatised in war zones or by awful events in their lives. Nor are we dismissive of efforts to help people who cannot, in the fullness of time, recover emotionally. However, our hearts sink every time we hear on the news that teams of counsellors have been sent in to the aftermath of a catastrophe. Not only is there evidence that psychological intervention can be harmful under these circumstances (Gerson and Olff 2005), but there is also a powerful message to society at large that recovery depends on the help of professionals, discouraging personal autonomy in the face of adversity. The legitimate role of mental health services is to help people overcome mental illness. Sadly, if Karl Marx were still alive, he might well conclude that medication and counselling, rather than religion, is now the opium of the people, stifling their drive to improve their situation for themselves. Like the purveyors of opium, the pharmaceutical industry, the psychotherapeutic establishment and organised psychiatry might have some difficulty in persuading him that their efforts at easing the pains of living are altruistic rather than self-serving.

No one has all the answers as far as treating mental illness is concerned. If any one treatment were substantially better than any other, then there would not be such a range of treatments available. However, individual practitioners tend to become very attached to a particular approach. Unfortunately, there is a tendency to join a faction, and then to exaggerate the advantages of one's own approach and to minimise the strengths of other approaches. This creates the caricature of the 'biological psychiatrist' and the 'psychotherapeutic psychiatrist'. One of us gave up regarding himself as a psychotherapeutic psychiatrist after a trainee told him: 'The things you talk about are much more interesting than Dr X (*avowedly biological psychiatrist*), but the things you do are exactly the same.'

In a world where the ultimate causes of mental illness are obscure, and where all treatments have significant drawbacks, it is only ethical and fair to patients to be clear and open about this. To claim otherwise, to assert that particular drugs or psychotherapies hold the solution to some or all mental health problems, is to become a charlatan.

. . . But Sometimes Helpful, Nonetheless

The divisions and disputes in the mental health community that have been so prominent in the past, lessen and intensify over time. In the background there is reasonable consensus that psychiatrists are necessary (which is reassuring). Those who want psychiatry abolished bolster their arguments through the creation of the straw man of the psychiatrist as bio-fanatic, a caricature of psychiatric practice that is incompatible with the content of this book. Social psychiatry has come back into fashion as a research area and as a paradigm. Professor Sir Robin Murray is a good scientist and after a lifetime of research as a biological psychiatrist, he has concluded that social factors are probably more important than biological factors in schizophrenia (BBC Radio 4, *The Life Scientific*, 7 February 2012, www.bbc.co.uk/programmes/b01bwmvt). The seemingly relentless advance of the 'biological revolution' in the USA shows clear signs of faltering, and disillusionment has set in over mono-therapeutic CBT (a historical error that is at risk of being repeated through wild over-enthusiasm for mindfulness based techniques).

Social psychiatry research tends to be large-scale and expensive, and it generates few commercial opportunities. It is difficult to get funding for it. However, social psychiatry is the dominant (though implicit) model for clinical psychiatrists in the UK, especially for those who work with deprived populations. There are a number of advantages to social psychiatry as a working model. It is pragmatic and eclectic. It does not demand membership of a tribe with an a priori belief in a particular casual model for mental illness. It is concerned with those factors that are realities in people's lives, rather than intangibles such as neurotransmitters or very rapid automatic thoughts outside of awareness. It can incorporate scientific advances without a paradigm shift, and it is as accessible to patients and families as it is to professionals, because you do not need years of scientific training to understand it.

There is a growing consensus amongst professionals, patients and carers (and even some policy-makers) as to what type of psychiatrist is most helpful. When you talk to patients, they are generally clear about what they want in a psychiatrist, and their requirements are not unreasonable. Oddly, zealous attachment to a particular approach is not one of the things they want, though competence definitely is.

It is clear that patients like psychiatrists who are straight-talking, open, warm and engaged. They like doctors who can talk to them without being patronising and without using jargon, and who involve them in decision-making. People like to be treated as autonomous adults, with dignity and respect. Patients tend to like team working if it involves consistent individuals, and tend not to want to see the psychiatrist as often as the psychiatrist wants to see them. People like to learn to manage their own problems, and often recognise that dependency, though comfortable, is damaging.

A lot of doctors like hospitals, and some older ones go misty eyed at the mention of the closed asylum in which they used to work. Very few patients have a similar attitude. In fact, what patients object to more than anything else is being treated in hospitals. Most patients would prefer to avoid admission if at all possible, and are delighted when you make efforts to manage acute episodes of illness in their own home.

Above all, people are generally incredibly forgiving of their psychiatrists when they make mistakes or have made a difficult decision such as to detain them. There are two things that make a big difference under these circumstances: the first is if you can say that you are sorry, even if you also have to acknowledge that under the same circumstances you would do the same thing again; the second is if the patient can understand why you did what you did, and see that you did your best.

Good psychiatrists bring their humanity to their work. This allows the patient to relate to another real human being, the dyad thus sharing not just human failings, but also human strengths. There is a penalty for the doctor, because being emotionally engaged with people suffering from mental illness is distressing. However, it is worthwhile, because it allows you to get alongside the patient, with a facilitative, not a dependent, relationship. It is this that allows the psychiatrist to assist, rather than impede, recovery.

References

Ackerman, P. T., Newton, J. E. O., McPherson, W. B., Jones, J. G. and Dykman, R. A. (1998). Prevalence of post-traumatic stress disorder and other psychiatric diagnoses in three groups of abused children (sexual, physical and both). *Child Abuse and Neglect*, **22**(8): 759–74.

American Psychiatric Association (2013). *Diagnostic and Statistical Manual of Mental Disorders* (5th edn.). Arlington: American Psychiatric Publishing.

Anthony, J. C., LeResche, L., Niaz, U., Von Korff, M. R. and Folstein, M. F. (1982). Limits of the 'Mini-Mental State' as a screening test for dementia and delirium among hospital patients. *Psychological Medicine*, **12**(2): 397–408.

Appleby, L., Kapur, N., Shaw, J., Windfuhr, K., Hunt, I. M. et al. (2015) *The National Confidential Inquiry into Suicide and Homicide by People with Mental Illness Annual Report 2015: England, Northern Ireland, Scotland and Wales*. University of Manchester. www.bbmh.manchester.ac.uk/cmhs/research/centreforsuicideprevention/nci/reports/NCISHReport2015Bookmarked3.pdf.

Bentall, R. P. (1992). A proposal to classify happiness as a psychiatric disorder. *Journal of Medical Ethics*, **18**(2): 94–98. (2003). *Madness Explained: Psychosis and Human Nature*. London: Allen Lane.

Bentall, R. P., Wickham, S., Shevlin, M. and Varese, F. (2012). Do specific early-life adversities lead to specific symptoms of psychosis? A study from the 2007 Adult Psychiatric Morbidity Study. *Schizophrenia Bulletin*, **38**: 734–40.

Brennan, P. A., Grekin, E. R. and Vanman, E. J. (2000). Major mental disorders and crime in the community. In *Violence among the Mentally Ill* (ed. P. Hodgins) (pp. 3–18). Dordrecht: Springer.

British Psychological Society (2013). *Division of Clinical Psychology Position Statement on the Classification of Behaviour and Experience in Relation to Functional Psychiatric Diagnoses: Time for a Paradigm Shift*. Leicester: BPS.

British Psychological Society Division of Clinical Psychology (2010). *The Core Purpose and Philosophy of the Profession*. Leicester: BPS.

Burns, T. (2013). *Our Necessary Shadow: The Nature and Meaning of Psychiatry*. London: Allen Lane.

Casey, P. and Kelly, B. (2007). *Fish's Clinical Psychopathology: Signs and Symptoms in Psychiatry* (3rd edn.). London: Royal College of Psychiatrists.

Cleckley, H. (1988). *The Mask of Sanity* (5th edn.). Augusta, GA: Emily S. Cleckley.

Cooper, J. E., Kendell, R. E., Gurland, B. J., Sharpe, L., Copeland, J. R. M. et al. (1972). *Psychiatric Diagnosis in New York and London*. Maudsley Monograph No. 20. London: Oxford University Press.

Cooper, P., Caulfield, M. and Mason, T. (2010). Developing a procedure to test for intoxication and mental capacity: the 'Under the Influence Test' pilot study. *Mental Health Nursing (Online)*, **30**(2): 9–13.

Craddock, N., Antebi, D., Attenburrow, M. J., Bailey, A., Carson, A. et al. (2008). Wake-up call for British psychiatry. *British Journal of Psychiatry*, **193**(1): 6–9.

Cutting, J. (1990). *The Right Cerebral Hemisphere and Psychiatric Disorders*. Oxford University Press.

Daalman, K., Boks, M. P., Diederen, K. M., de Weijer, A. D., Blom, J. D. et al. (2011). The same or different? A phenomenological comparison of auditory verbal hallucinations in healthy and psychotic individuals. *Journal of Clinical Psychiatry*, **72**(3): 320–5.

David, A., Fleminger, S., Kopelman, M., Lovenstone, S. and Mellers, J. (2009). *Lishman's Organic Psychiatry: A Textbook of Neuropsychiatry* (4th edn.). Chichester: Wiley-Blackwell.

Douglas, K. S., Hart, S. D., Webster, C. D. and Belfrage, H. (2013). *HCR-20V3: Assessing Risk of Violence – User Guide.* Burnaby, BC: Mental Health, Law, and Policy Institute, Simon Fraser University.

Durkheim, E. (1951). *Suicide: A Study in Sociology* (ed. G. Simpson and J. A. Spaulding). New York: Free Press.

Edwards, G. and Gross, M. M. (1976). Alcohol dependence: provisional description of a clinical syndrome. *British Medical Journal,* **1**(6017): 1058–61.

Fink, M. and Taylor, M. A. (2003). *Catatonia: A Clinician's Guide to Diagnosis and Treatment.* Cambridge University Press.

Fish, F. and Hamilton, M. (1985). *Clinical Psychopathology* (2nd edn.). Bristol: Wright.

General Medical Council (2013). *Good Medical Practice.* London: GMC. www.gmc-uk.org/guidance/good_medical_practice/duties_of_a_doctor.asp.

Gerson, B. P. R. and Olff, M. (2005). Coping with the aftermath of trauma: authors' reply. *British Medical Journal,* **331**(7507): 50.

Hare, R. D. (1991).*The Hare Psychopathy Checklist – Revised.* Toronto: Multi-Health Systems.

Hert, M., Correll, C. U., Bobes, J., Cetkovich-Bakmas, M. A., Cohen, D. A. et al. (2011). Physical illness in patients with severe mental disorders. I. Prevalence, impact of medications and disparities in health care. *World Psychiatry,* **10**(1): 52–77.

Hollyman, J. A. and Hemsi, L. (1983). What do the examiners understand by formulation? *Psychiatric Bulletin,* **7**(9): 165–6.

Jaspers, K. (1913). *Allgemeine Psychopathologie.* Berlin: Springer.

Kavanagh, D. H., Tansey, K. E., O'Donovan, M. C. and Owen, M. J. (2015). Schizophrenia genetics: emerging themes for a complex disorder. *Molecular Psychiatry,* **20**(1): 72–6.

Kendell, R. E. (1976). The classification of depression: a review of contemporary confusion. *British Journal of Psychiatry,* **129**(1): 15–28.

Kevles, D. J. (1999). Eugenics and human rights. *British Medical Journal,* **319**(7207): 435–8.

Kinderman, P. (2014). *A Prescription for Psychiatry: Why We Need a Whole New Approach to Mental Health and Wellbeing.* Basingstoke: Palgrave Macmillan.

Komuravelli, A., Poole. R. and Higgo, R. (2011). Stability of the diagnosis of first-episode drug-induced psychosis. *The Psychiatrist,* **35**(6): 224–7.

Krawiecka, M., Goldberg, D. and Vaughan, M. (1977). A standardised psychiatric assessment scale for rating chronic psychotic patients. *Acta Psychiatrica Scandinavica,* **55**(4): 299–308.

Laing, R. D. (1990). *The Divided Self: An Existential Study in Sanity and Madness.* London: Penguin.

Lifton, R. J. (2000). *The Nazi Doctors: Medical Killing and the Psychology of Genocide.* New York: Basic Books.

Lishman, W. A. (1997). *Organic Psychiatry: The Psychological Consequences of Cerebral Disorder.* Oxford: Blackwell Science.

Lonie, J. A., Tierney, K. M. and Ebmeier, K. P. (2009). Screening for mild cognitive impairment: a systematic review. *International Journal of Geriatric Psychiatry,* **24**(9): 902–15.

Oyebode, F. (2015). *Sims' Symptoms in the Mind* (5th edn.). London: Saunders.

Poole, R. (2015). Emergencies involving alcohol. In *Emergency Psychiatry* (ed. K. Nicholls) (pp. 51–68). London: RCPsych Publications.

Poole, R. and Cook, C. (2011). Praying with a patient constitutes a breach of professional boundaries in psychiatric practice. *British Journal of Psychiatry,* **199**(2): 94–8.

Poole, R. and Higgo, R. (2011). Spirituality and the threat to therapeutic boundaries in psychiatric practice. *Mental Health, Religion and Culture,* **14**(1): 19–29.

Poole, R., Higgo, R. and Robinson, C. A. (2014). *Mental Health and Poverty.* Cambridge University Press.

Professional Affairs Board of the British Psychological Society (2000). *Learning Disability: Definitions and Contexts.* Leicester: British Psychological Society. www.bps.org.uk/system/files/documents/ppb_learning.pdf.

Rahman, R. S., Gupta, S., While, D., Rodway, R., Ibrahim, S. et al. (2013). *Quality of Risk Assessment Prior to*

Suicide and Homicide: A Pilot Study. National Confidential Inquiry into Suicide and Homicide by People with Mental Illness. University of Manchester.

Ritchie, J., Dick, D. and Lingham, R. (1994). *Report of the Inquiry into the Care and Treatment of Christopher Clunis.* North East Thames and South East Thames Regional Health Authority: HMSO.

Romme, M. and Escher, S. (eds.) (1993). *Accepting Voices.* London: MIND Publications.

Royal College of Psychiatrists (2014). *Good Practice in the Management of Autism (including Asperger Syndrome) in Adults.* College Report CR191. London: RCPsych. www.rcpsych.ac.uk/usefulresources/publi cations/collegereports/cr/cr191.aspx.

Schneider, K. (1959). *Clinical Psychopathology.* New York: Grune and Stratton.

Shevlin, M., Dorahy, M. and Adamson, G. (2007). Childhood traumas and hallucinations: an analysis of the National Co-Morbidity Survey. *Journal of Psychiatric Research,* **41**: 222–8.

Summerfield, D. (2001). The invention of post-traumatic stress disorder and the social usefulness of a psychiatric category. *British Medical Journal,* **322**(7278): 95–8.

Taylor, P. J. and Gunn, J. (1999). Homicides by people with mental illness: myth and reality. *British Journal of Psychiatry,* **174**(1): 9–14.

Van Os, J., Hanssen, M., Bijl, R. V. and Ravelli, A. (2000). Strauss (1969) revisited: a psychosis continuum in the general population? *Schizophrenia Research,* **45**(1): 11–20.

World Health Organization (1992). *Classification of Mental and Behavioural Disorders: Clinical Descriptions and Diagnostic Guidelines* (10th edn.). Geneva: WHO.

(2003). Adult ADHD Self-Report Scale-V1.1 (ASRS-V1.1). Symptoms Checklist from WHO Composite International Diagnostic Interview. Geneva: WHO. www.hcp.med.harvard.edu/ncs/ftpdir/ adhd/18Q_ASRS_English.pdf.

(2016). International Statistical Classification of Diseases and Related Health Problems 10th Revision (ICD-10)-WHO Version for 2016. Geneva: WHO. http:// apps.who.int/classifications/icd10/ browse/2016/en#/F60-F69.

Zigmond, A. S. and Snaith, R. P. (1983). The hospital anxiety and depression scale. *Acta Psychiatrica Scandinavica,* **67**(6): 361–70

Index